E.I. Hernández-Jiménez, E.M. Rakhanskaya

MICROCURRENT, ULTRASOUND, AND LED THERAPY
IN COSMETIC DERMATOLOGY & SKINCARE PRACTICE

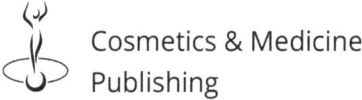
Cosmetics & Medicine Publishing

Author:
Elena I. Hernández-Jiménez, *Ph.D.*

Editor:
Ekaterina M. Rakhanskaya, *M.D.* Neurologist, radiation safety specialist

MICROCURRENT, ULTRASOUND, AND LED THERAPY IN COSMETIC DERMATOLOGY AND SKINCARE PRACTICE

When people talk about aesthetic devices, they primarily mean high-energy technologies such as lasers, intense pulsed light (IPL), high-intensity focused ultrasound (HIFU), radio frequency (RF), etc., but this unfairly overlooks low-energy therapy. Low-energy devices (referred to as cosmetic devices) are the most widespread in skincare practice. If you understand how they work, they can be used to achieve aesthetic results that are just as significant as those produced by high-energy devices. We created this book to explain how the most popular non-invasive skincare methods — modern low-energy microcurrent, ultrasound (US), and light-emitting diode (LED) therapy — work.

In our book, there are no duty words from leaflets, which you can find in many manual guides for devices. We have collected scientifically valid information about all these methods. Only by understanding how they act can you achieve the best results.

We explain simply and in detail what electricity, ultrasound (US), and light are and how they affect the skin. We discuss which parameters are essential and which are just marketing claims. We tell you what results can be achieved with microcurrent, US therapy and peeling, sonophoresis, and LED therapy, as well as what you should not expect from these approaches and what technologies they should be distinguished from. In addition, we cover the increasingly popular plasma therapy — exposure of the skin to low-temperature plasma (so-called cold plasma). Everything you need to know about these devices and methods to understand them and perform effective treatments is in this book.

ISBN 978-1-970196-20-7 (paperback)
ISBN 978-1-970196-41-2 (hardcover)
ISBN 978-1-970196-10-8 (eBook – Adobe PDF)
ISBN 978-1-970196-19-1 (eBook – ePUB)

© Cosmetics & Medicine Publishing LLC, 2024
© Cover photo: Evgeny Varlamov / Shutterstock

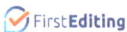

English version is edited and certified by the FirstEditing.Com, Inc. (USA).

Author

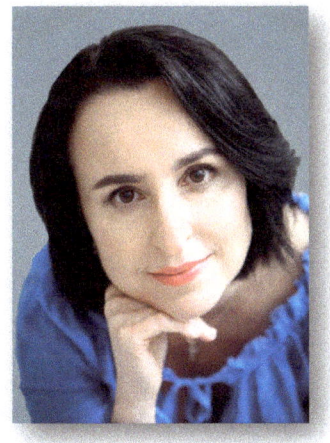

Elena I. Hernández-Jiménez, *Ph.D.*

Biophysicist, scientific journalist

Editor-in-chief of Cosmetics and Medicine Publishing

Chairperson of the Executive Board of the International Society of Applied Corneotherapy (I.A.C.)

Author and co-author of numerous publications in professional magazines, co-author and editor of the book series *Fundamentals of Cosmetic Dermatology & Skincare*, *Cosmetic Dermatology & Skincare Practice*, Cosmetic *Chemistry for Dermatology & Skincare Specialists* and others

Speaker at international conferences, author of training seminars and webinars for professionals in the field of skincare

Professional interests: biology and physiology of the skin, skin permeability, cosmetic chemistry, anti-age medicine, physiotherapy in dermatology and aesthetic medicine, skin analysis and imaging

Table of Contents

Abbreviations. 8
Introduction 9

PART I
MICROCURRENT THERAPY

Chapter 1. The nature of electricity 11
1.1. Electricity and electric current 11
1.2. Main parameters of electric current determining
its interaction with the body 15
   1.2.1. Intensity of exposure (electric current, voltage) 15
   1.2.2. Direct and alternating electric current 16
   1.2.3. Continuous and pulsed current 16
   1.2.4. Exposure duration 17

Chapter 2. Effects of electric current on the body 18
2.1. Electric current-related effects 18
   2.1.1. Changes in the quantitative and qualitative ratio of ions . . . 19
   2.1.2. Increased ion activity in tissues. 19
   2.1.3. Electric polarization 19
   2.1.4. Changes in the acid–base balance (pH) 20
   2.1.5. Electroosmosis 20
   2.1.6. Heating 20
2.2. Peculiarities of the effect of current on the skin 21
2.3. History of electrotherapy 24
2.4. Variety of electrotherapy methods 28

Chapter 3. Microcurrent therapy 31
3.1. Principle of microcurrent action 31

3.2. Microcurrent therapy parameters 33
3.3. Effects of microcurrent therapy 34
3.4. Indications 36
3.5. Contraindications 37
3.6. Microcurrent therapy devices 38
3.7. Microcurrent therapy treatment specifics 40
3.8. Transcutaneous electroneurostimulation, dynamic
     electroneurostimulation 40
3.9. What microcurrent therapy should be distinguished from 42
    3.9.1. Galvanization 42
    3.9.2. Iontophoresis 44
    3.9.3. Desincrustation 47
    3.9.4. Diadynamic therapy 47
    3.9.5. Diadynamophoresis 49
    3.9.6. Electromyostimulation 49
    3.9.7. Electrolypolysis 49

Chapter 4. Plasma therapy 51
4.1. The nature of plasma 51
4.2. Biomedical effects of plasma and plasma
     technology options 53
4.3. Indications 57

PART II
ULTRASOUND THERAPY

Chapter 1. The nature of ultrasound 59
1.1. Sound wave generation and propagation in matter 59
1.2. Ultrasound parameters determining the interaction
     with living tissues 60
    1.2.1. Frequency of sound vibrations 60
    1.2.2. Amplitude and intensity 61
    1.2.3. Acoustic impedance 62

Chapter 2. Ultrasound action on the body and skin ... 64
2.1. Mechanical impact. ... 64
2.2. Physicochemical impact ... 65
2.3. Thermal effect ... 66
2.4. Reflex effects. ... 67
2.5. Non-thermal effects ... 67

Chapter 3. Low-energy ultrasound techniques ... 69
3.1. Local ultrasound therapy. ... 69
    3.1.1. Biological and clinical effects ... 69
    3.1.2. Indications for local ultrasound therapy ... 72
3.2. Ultrasonic peeling ... 72
    3.2.1. Biological and clinical effects ... 72
    3.2.2. Indications. ... 73
    3.2.3. Features of ultrasonic peeling ... 73
3.3. Sonophoresis (phonophoresis) ... 75
    3.3.1. Basic parameters of sonophoresis ... 77
    3.3.2. Mechanisms for increasing the skin permeability ... 78
    3.3.3. Sonophoresis protocols. ... 82
    3.3.4. Opportunities and limitations ... 83

PART III

LED THERAPY (PHOTOBIOMODULATION)

Chapter 1. The nature of light ... 87
1.1. Light and its parameters ... 87
1.2. Laser devices. ... 89
    1.2.1. How lasers work ... 90
    1.2.2. Laser types ... 92
1.3. Basic parameters of laser radiation that determine laser–target interactions ... 94
    1.3.1. Wavelength of the generated radiation ... 94
    1.3.2. Energy density (fluence) and power ... 96
    1.3.3. Laser operating mode: pulsed or continuous ... 97
    1.3.4. Light spot and energy focusing ... 97

Chapter 2. Interaction of laser radiation with the skin 98
2.1. Laser targets 98
2.2. Laser exposure mechanisms 99

Chapter 3. Photobiomodulation 102
3.1. Low laser (light) therapy mechanisms of action 104
    3.1.1. Mitochondrial hypothesis 105
    3.1.2. Oxidative stress hypothesis 106
    3.1.3. Copper hypothesis 107
    3.1.4. Thermodynamic hypothesis 107
3.2. Clinical effects and therapeutic applications 110
3.3. Indications and applications in skincare 115
    3.3.1. Age-related skin changes 115
    3.3.2. Skin recovery 116
    3.3.3. Acne 116
    3.3.4. Pigmentation disorders: vitiligo and pigment lesions 117
    3.3.5. Atopic dermatitis and psoriasis 118
    3.3.6. Alopecia 118
    3.3.7. Local fat deposits 119
3.4. Contraindications 120

Afterword 121
References 122

Abbreviations

α-SMA	— smooth muscle alpha-actin	LTR	— localized transport region
AP-1	— activating protein 1	MitMP	— mitochondrial membrane potential
ATP	— adenosine triphosphate	MMP	— matrix metalloproteinase
bFGF	— basic fibroblast growth factor	Nd:YAG	— neodymium-doped yttrium-aluminum-garnet laser
CMW	— centimeter wave		
CNS	— central nervous system	NF-κB	— nuclear factor kappa B
Cu-GHK	— copper-containing tripeptide glycyl-L-histidyl-L-lysine	NMR	— nuclear magnetic resonance
		NO	— nitric oxide
DENS	— dynamic electric neurostimulation	PDL	— pulsed dye laser
DMW	— decimeter wave	pH	— pondus Hydrogenii
DNA	— deoxyribonucleic acid	RF	— radio frequency
EMS	— electromyostimulation	ROS	— reactive oxygen species
Er:YAG	— erbium-doped yttrium-aluminum-garnet laser	SI	— International Systems of Units
GaAlAs	— gallium-aluminum arsenide	SOD	— superoxide dismutase
		TENS	— transcutaneous electrical nerve stimulation
GaAs	— gallium arsenide		
HeNe	— xenon–neon	TGF-β	— transforming growth factor beta
HFS	— high-frequency sonophoresis	TIMP	— tissue inhibitor of metalloproteinases
HIFU	— high-intensity focused ultrasound	TNF-α	— tumor necrosis factor alpha
HSP	— heat shock proteins		
IL	— interleukin	UHF	— ultra-high frequency
IPL	— intense pulsed light	US	— ultrasound
IR	— infrared	UV	— ultraviolet
KTP	— potassium titanyl phosphate laser	UVA	— ultraviolet type A
		UVB	— ultraviolet type B
LED	— light-emitting diode	UVC	— ultraviolet type C
LFS	— low-frequency sonophoresis	XeCl	— xenon–chlorine
		XeF	— xenon–fluorine
LLLT	— low-level laser (light) therapy		

Introduction

When people talk about aesthetic devices, they primarily mean high-energy technologies such as laser, intense pulsed light (IPL), high-intensity focused ultrasound (HIFU), radio frequency (RF), etc. However, this overlooks low-energy therapy, which also aims to rejuvenate, restore, and revitalize the skin, just in a different way. High-energy devices destroy the skin so that, in place of the damaged "defective" skin, our body builds a new "healthy" skin. Low-energy methods stimulate various processes in the skin, which helps to improve its structure and functioning.

That's why we dedicated one of the books in the *Cosmetic Dermatology & Skincare* series to the most popular low-energy microcurrent, ultrasound (US) and light-emitting diode (LED) therapy devices. While these devices are actively used in almost all beauty salons and aesthetic clinics, not all practitioners understand how they work. Yet, this understanding is crucial for the most effective and safe treatments.

Part I

Microcurrent therapy

Chapter 1
The nature of electricity

There is practically no phenomenon in nature that is not accompanied by electricity.

Richard Feynman,
Nobel Prize Laureate in Physics, 1965

To understand how microcurrent acts on the human body, we first need to know what electricity is. Let's try to break this question down into simple terms.

1.1. Electricity and electric current

Back in high school physics, we were told that **electric current** is a directed (ordered) movement of charged particles, i.e., particles that have an electric charge. So what are these charged particles?

These are negatively charged **electrons** and positively charged **protons**. Positrons, antiprotons, and discrete quark charges are also charged particles, but these are short-lived particles worth discussing only in terms of quantum physics and not in the framework of this book.

In the stable form, atoms or molecules have a neutral charge (that is, the number of protons in the atomic nuclei equals the number of electrons in their orbitals), but due to various processes, electrons can break away and exist in a free form. Alternatively, a neutral molecule may "divide" into a part in which there are more electrons (negatively charged ion, anion) and a part in which there are not enough electrons to compensate for the positive charge of the protons (positively charged ion, cation) (**Fig. I-1-1**). In general, an **ion** is a particle (atom or molecule) with an electric charge. Thus, single ions (atomic or molecular) and multi-atomic ion complexes (dust particles, droplets, etc.) can be charge carriers.

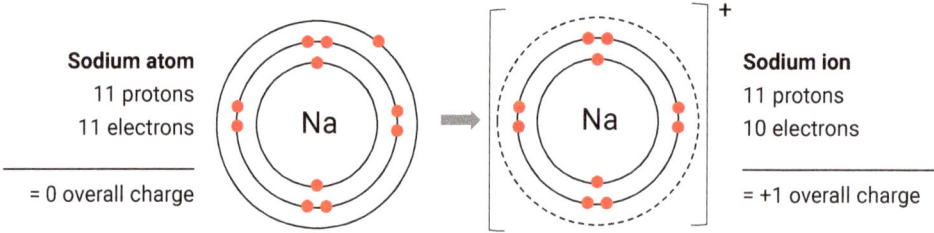

Figure I-1-1. Schematic of the differences between the neutral sodium atom and the positively (+1) charged sodium ion

Some materials have many such charge carriers (or they can easily arise under the influence of an external electric field); these are called **conductors**. Materials in which there are few charge carriers (or particles that can become such under the influence of an electric field) are called **dielectrics** — materials that are relatively poor conductors of electric current.

Metals are the best conductors of electricity. They are also called Type 1 conductors because their main charge carriers are electrons. Solutions or molten electrolytes (Type 2 conductors) with ions as charge carriers are also good conductors. Gases under ordinary conditions conduct electricity poorly. They are referred to as dielectrics, but they also contain ions and electrons, the concentration of which may significantly increase under certain conditions. There are also so-called **semiconductors** — materials whose ability to conduct electric current is between that of conductors and dielectrics but increases significantly with increasing temperature and exposure to various kinds of radiation. The charge carriers in semiconductors are electrons and holes (so-called quasiparticles — positive charge carriers formed in the absence of electrons migrating from one atom to another).

What makes these charged particles move in an orderly fashion (because under normal conditions, this movement is chaotic)? In other words, what generates an electric current (**Fig. I-1-2**)?

An electric current can arise:
- Due to an **external electric field** formed by current sources. Most often, these devices convert different types of energy into electrical energy. In these sources, electric charges are separated so that the positive and negative charges are accumulated at the oppo-

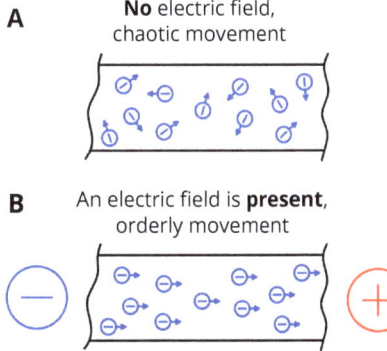

Figure I-1-2. Movement of electrons: a — in the absence of an external electric field, B — in its presence

site poles, resulting in the so-called **potential difference**. In everyday life, the simplest example of current sources are batteries with opposite poles. Medical devices usually have reversely charged electrodes delivering electric current to the human body. The positive electrode is called an **anode** and the negative electrode is a **cathode**.

When the electrodes come into contact with a conductor, the electrical circuit is closed and the charged particles of the conductor begin moving toward the electrode with the opposite charge in an orderly manner. Thus, an electric current occurs when there is a potential difference between the two points of the conductor. On one side, there is a negative charge and on the other side, there is a positive charge. An important condition is the presence of a closed circuit, i.e., a single space that creates conditions for the orderly movement of charged particles.

- When **conductors are heated** (because increasing the temperature of conductors increases the number of charge carriers), electrons become more mobile and can bounce off atoms. If you heat one part of a conductor and cool the other, there will also be a potential difference between them and, therefore, a current will flow.
- **During various chemical reactions**, which will also result in the formation of charge carriers and, consequently, potential differences between different conductor poles.
- **Under exposure to a magnetic field.** An alternating electric current forms a magnetic field, which can form an electric field, i.e., a potential difference.

In turn, the very orderly motion of charged particles (electric current) can lead to the following phenomena:
- heating (observed in all conductors except superconductors) due to friction

- changes in the chemical composition observed mainly in electrolytes due to electrolysis
- creation of a magnetic field (observed in all conductors without exception)

Terms & Definitions

- **Electric field** is created by electric charges and charged particles in space.
- **Magnetic field** is created by the movement of electric charges along a conductor.
- **Electromagnetic field** is a special form of matter through which the interaction between electrically charged particles (electrons, ions) occurs. The field can be viewed as the combination of an electric field and a magnetic field. The electric field is produced by stationary charges, and the magnetic field by moving charges (electric currents); these two are often described as the sources of the field. Continuously changing, both components maintain the existence of the electromagnetic field.
- The field of a stationary or moving particle is inextricably linked to the carrier (charged particle). However, during the accelerated motion of carriers, the electromagnetic field from them "tears off" and exists (propagates) in the environment independently, in the form of an **electromagnetic wave**, not disappearing with the elimination of the carrier. For example, radio waves do not disappear when the electric current (electrons) disappears from the antenna that radiates them.
- **Light** is also electromagnetic radiation; most commonly, light is understood as the visible part of the electromagnetic spectrum. We see electromagnetic waves in the visible light range thanks to our eyes and brain, which perceive the waves as colored depending on the wavelength. In medicine, the term "light" refers to the entire optical range of the electromagnetic spectrum: ultraviolet (UV), visible, and infrared (IR) radiation.
- A **wave** (in general) is a disturbance in the medium (as for sound) or field (different types of electromagnetic oscillations), which propagates in space with a finite speed.

1.2. Main parameters of electric current determining its interaction with the body

1.2.1. Intensity of exposure (electric current, voltage)

When we describe the effect of any type of energy, the first thing we are interested in is the intensity, which largely determines the resulting effects. However, to describe the effects correctly, it is necessary to consider not only the amount of energy but also other parameters that will characterize the features of interaction of a given physical factor with a target. This is relevant both for electric current and for ultrasound and light effects.

In the case of electricity, the main quantitative measure of exposure is the **electric current**, i.e., the ratio of the amount of electricity (moving charged particles, electrons, etc.) that passes through the cross-section of the conductor to the time of its passage.

The reason that we can't characterize the electric current only by the amount of electricity (the number of charged particles) is that the same amount of charge carriers can pass through a large or small conductor (imagine affecting a mouse and a person), for a second or for an hour, and therefore provoke completely different effects in the conductor.

The International System of Units (SI) uses the **Ampere (A)** as the unit for measuring electric current. One Ampere is equal to 1 Coulomb, or $6.241509074 \times 10^{18}$ electrons worth of charge, moving past a point in a second.

Another parameter that reflects the intensity of the electric current is **voltage**, which is the potential difference between two points in an electric circuit. In other words, it is the pressure from an electric circuit's power source that pushes charged electrons (current) through a conducting loop. If we use the well-known analogy of electric current with the water flow, the intensity of electric current describes the amount of water that flows, and the voltage is the pressure that makes the water move; the higher it is, the faster the water flows. The unit of voltage is the **Volt (V)**.

1.2.2. Direct and alternating electric current

A direct electric current flows in one direction; at a low voltage and low strength, it is called **galvanic**.

An alternating current occurs when the flow of charged particles reverses direction at a given frequency. This frequency is expressed in **Hertz (Hz)**, the SI unit equivalent to one event (or cycle) per second. Depending on the frequency, alternating currents can be classed as:
- Low frequency: up to 1000 Hz
- Medium frequency: 1–10 kHz
- High frequency: above 10 kHz

1.2.3. Continuous and pulsed current

The flow of charged particles may occur continuously, or it may occur in certain portions. Such a current is called pulsed. a pulsed current can be both direct current (flowing in one direction) and alternating current (changing direction with a certain frequency, see section 1.2.2 above).

The **frequency of the pulses** is determined by the frequency at which the current is switched on and off. It is also measured in Hertz.

The **shape of the pulses** is an important parameter that determines the features of energy delivery. In general, all pulses have three parts: (1) the initial rise, which characterizes the peculiarities of switching on the electric circuit, (2) the top, which can be flat or curved and which reflects the supply of peak energy levels, and (3) the cut, which is the final voltage drop. The following pulses may occur:
- Rectangular — current intensity instantly reaches maximum values, stays at the same level for some time, and disappears instantly
- Triangular — the current intensity gradually reaches a maximum and then decreases to zero
- Bell-shaped — the current intensity increases rapidly at first, then slows down, reaching its maximum, and then decreases in the same way
- Sawtooth-like — similar to triangular, but either the rise or fall of the current intensity is instantaneous, while the other "facet" is gradual

- Trapezoidal — like rectangular, but the rise and fall of the current intensity occur gradually, not instantaneously
- Exponential — a smooth rise of current up to the maximum followed by a smooth decrease, especially towards the end of the pulse, etc.

1.2.4. Exposure duration

This is an important parameter that, along with other parameters, determines the degree of the effects. The electrotherapy treatment protocols always indicate the exposure time and always follow the recommendations of the manufacturer of the device used.

Chapter 2
Effects of electric current on the body

Who would have thought that electric current, to the point of being so weak that it could not be detected even by the most sensitive electrometers, is capable of acting with such force on the organs of the animal…

Alessandro Volta

Electrotherapy is a part of physical therapy based on dosed exposure of the body to electric currents and electric, magnetic, or electromagnetic fields.

This aspect of physical therapy is the most extensive and includes methods based on the use of direct and alternating currents of varying frequencies and pulse shapes.

Recall that magnetic and electric fields do not exist in isolation from each other, but one may predominate. When the proportions are comparable, we refer to an electromagnetic field propagating in space as electromagnetic waves. Therefore, magnetotherapy is a part of electrotherapy which uses magnetic fields for therapeutic purposes.

2.1. Electric current-related effects

The main conductors of electric current in the body are electrolytes — salts, acids, and alkalis capable of dissociating into ions in solution. Their motion determines the primary effect of electric current on the body, although the effects of different types of current (direct and alternating, high-frequency and low-frequency, etc.) will differ.

There are several physicochemical shifts that the passage of current can provoke. These trigger further changes in the cells and tissues underlying the clinical results.

2.1.1. Changes in the quantitative and qualitative ratio of ions

Changing the quantitative and qualitative ratio of ions is the most essential process. Due to the differences in ions (charge, size, degree of hydration, etc.) the speed of their movement in tissues will differ.

For example, after galvanization (exposure to a direct current of constant intensity), a pronounced ionic asymmetry occurs in the tissues, which affects the vital activity of cells. a characteristic manifestation of ionic asymmetry is the relative predominance of univalent cations (K^+, Na^+) at the cathode and divalent cations (Ca^{2+}, Mg^{2+}) at the anode.

2.1.2. Increased ion activity in tissues

This phenomenon is caused by the transition of a part of ions from the state bound with polyelectrolytes (in particular, proteins) into the free form. This contributes to the increase in the physiological activity of tissues and is considered one of the mechanisms of the biostimulation effect of electric current.

2.1.3. Electric polarization

Electric polarization is the accumulation of oppositely charged ions near cell membranes with the formation of an electromotive force that has a direction opposite to the applied voltage. This phenomenon is the most essential among the primary mechanisms of direct current action.

Polarization changes cell membrane permeability and affects the diffusion of many compounds, including water. a cascade of reactions characteristic of reversible cell damage is initiated, causing the synthesis of heat shock proteins (HSPs) to be stimulated in the cells. Although polarization itself fades within a few hours, a mechanism of nonspecific adaptation is triggered in the cells, which enhances the reparation potential of tissues.

2.1.4. Changes in the acid–base balance (pH)

Changes in the acid–base balance in tissues due to the movement of positive hydrogen ions to the cathode and negative hydroxyl ions to the anode are among the physicochemical effects of galvanization. Changes in tissue pH* affect the activity of enzymes, tissue respiration, and the state of biocolloids, and serve as a source of irritation of skin receptors.

2.1.5. Electroosmosis

Since the ions are hydrated — that is, covered with a water "coat" — along with the movement of ions during galvanization, there is a movement of liquid (water) in the direction of the cathode (this phenomenon is called electroosmosis). Consequently, under the cathode, there is edema and loosening, and there is tissue shrinking and tightening around the anode, which should be considered, especially when treating inflammatory processes. These and other physicochemical effects of galvanic current determine its physiological and therapeutic impact.

2.1.6. Heating

Above, we have named the effects induced directly by the current passage. However, the peculiarities of its flow will depend not only on the characteristics of the electric current itself but also on the medium (in our case, body tissues) through which it passes. These features are

---

* pH (lat. *pondus Hydrogenii*) is a quantitative measure of the acidity or basicity of aqueous or other liquid solutions. Measured on a scale of 0 to 14. a pH value of 7 is neutral, which means it is neither acidic nor basic. a pH value of less than 7 means it is more acidic, and a pH value of more than 7 means it is more basic.

reflected in Ohm's law, which defines the relationship between voltage **(V)** and current **(I)** via electrical resistance **(R)** — the current in a circuit is directly proportional to the voltage and inversely proportional to resistance:

$$I = U / R$$

Electrical resistance characterizes the ability of a medium (electrical conductor) to prevent the passage of electric current. It is essentially the inverse of the electrical conductivity of the material.

Obviously, the passage of charge carriers through the medium is not free because they interact with other structures. The movement of charged particles during current passage through tissues is accompanied by their collision with each other, as well as with tissue components. This results in the **generation of heat**, which affects the course of a variety of processes in cells and tissues and largely determines the effect of various electrotherapeutic methods on the body. **With direct and pulsed currents, heat is generated insignificantly, while high-frequency alternating currents cause a considerable amount of heat in the tissues, leading to vascular reactions and changes in blood supply.**

The higher the electrical resistance, the more electrical energy is lost due to the internal resistance of the conductive medium. The unit of the electrical resistance measured with direct current is the **Ohm (Ω)**.

Although different materials have different resistance, it can vary greatly depending on the cross-section, temperature, magnitude, and frequency of the current.

2.2. Peculiarities of the effect of current on the skin

Undamaged human skin with the intact *stratum corneum* has high ohmic resistance and low specific conductivity; therefore, current penetrates the body mainly through the outlet ducts of sweat and sebaceous glands and intercellular gaps containing electrolytes. Since the total area of pores does not exceed 1/200 of the skin surface, most of the current energy is spent on overcoming the *stratum corneum*, which has the greatest resistance. The "living" layers of the epidermis under the *stratum corneum* and the dermis are rich in water, so their electrical resistance to current is low. However, subcutaneous fatty tissue, which has a lot of lipids, is a poor conductor of electric current. Having overcome the resistance of *stratum corneum* and subcutaneous adipose tissue, the current is further distributed mainly through intercellular spaces, muscles, blood, and lymphatic vessels, deviating significantly from the straight line which can conditionally connect two electrodes. To a lesser extent, direct current passes through nerves, tendons, adipose tissue, and bones. Electric current practically does not pass through nails, hair, or the *stratum corneum* of dry skin.

Skin conductivity depends on many factors, primarily on water–electrolyte balance. Thus, tissues with hyperemia and/or edema are characterized by higher conductivity than healthy ones.

Electric current can lead to the redistribution of ions and water in the affected skin area, causing local changes in the acidity of the extracellular microenvironment and edema. Redistribution of ions can affect the membrane potential of cells, changing their functional activity, such as by stimulating a mild stress response leading to the synthesis of protective HSPs.

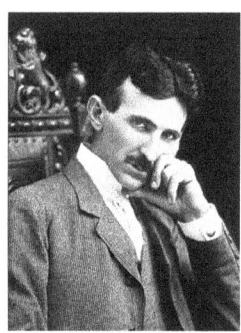

Nikola Tesla
(1856–1943)

We should also say a few words about high-frequency electrotherapy, of which Nikola Tesla can be considered the pioneer. He introduced this idea in his speech to the American Electrotherapy Association in Buffalo on September 13, 1898: "One of the recently noted and surprising features of high-frequency currents which has mainly interested physicians has proved to be their complete harmlessness to man, allowing a comparatively large amount of electrical energy to pass through the human body without causing pain or serious discomfort."

The main active factor of all high-frequency methods is an alternating current, either brought directly to the patient's body or generated in tissues and body environments under the influence of alternating electromagnetic fields of high and ultrahigh frequency.

The basis of the physiological and therapeutic impact of high-frequency vibrations is their interaction with the charged particles of biological tissues, which include not only ions, but also proteins, low-molecular-weight metabolites, polar heads of phospholipids, and nucleic acids. Since the above-mentioned charged molecules have different sizes, their motion will occur at different resonance frequencies.

As we know, **resonance is observed when the frequency of natural vibrations of structures coincides with the frequency of the acting physical factor**. An example of resonance is the ringing of crystal glasses caused by high-frequency sounds during singing. From the point of view of physics, molecules in a cell can be represented as oscillating systems (oscillators) like a ball on a spring. Each oscillating molecule has its strictly defined oscillation frequency or, if the oscillator is asymmetric, its frequency spectrum. Variable electric and electromagnetic fields can rock the molecules and supply energy in portions; in other words, they bring them into resonance until the vibrational energy exceeds the binding energy of the molecule. Absorption of resonant oscillations is accompanied by two types of effects: non-specific (thermal) and specific (non-thermal, or oscillatory). On the surface of membranes and possibly macromolecules there are layers of unmixed water, which can significantly reduce the permeability of biomembranes and slow down the interaction of macromolecules with enzymes. The impact of high-frequency vibrations on water molecules can destroy such "water coats" around membranes and biopolymers, thus accelerating many physiologically important processes.

Under the action of high-frequency fields, oscillations and collisions of free current carriers occur, which in living tissues are ions. This effect is the basis of the conduction current. The molecule can be neutral, but it will have charges at its ends (they will cancel each other, resulting in zero total charge). Such a molecule, called a **dipole**, will rotate in an alternating field, generating heat. The amount of generated heat depends both on the parameters of the acting factor (current intensity, frequency) and on the electrical properties of the tissues themselves. Therefore, high-frequency therapy is selective in nature.

In practice, this means that, by changing the frequency, it is possible to achieve selective heating of certain tissues. Since the heating of tissues is caused by the absorption of certain resonant frequencies, it is carried out from inside, and the sensitive sensors on the skin do not feel the heat. An increase in tissue temperature is accompanied by hyperemia, increased permeability of blood–tissue barriers and microcirculation, and stimulation of metabolic processes.

2.3. History of electrotherapy

Electrotherapy was born in 1780 thanks to the visionary eye of Lucia Galeazzi — wife of Luigi Galvani and daughter of his teacher. It was Lucia's job to turn the handle of an electroforming machine while an assistant dissected a frog under Galvani's supervision. The frog's foot was beating under the scalpel, and the observant woman noticed that cramps occurred when a spark leaped between the balls of the machine. She drew her husband's attention to this coincidence, and the revolution in physics that gave birth to the doctrine of the role of electricity in the functioning of living systems began.

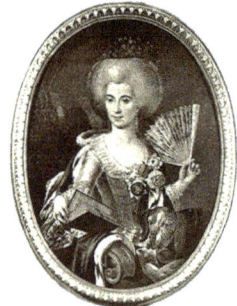

Lucia Galeazzi
(1743–1788)

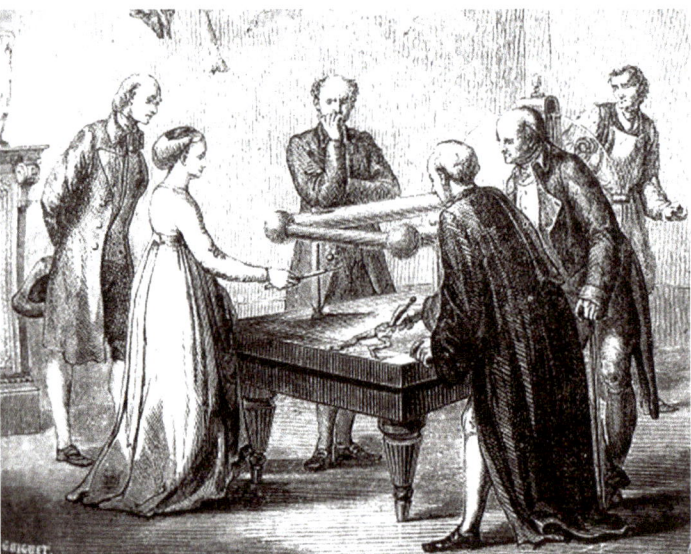

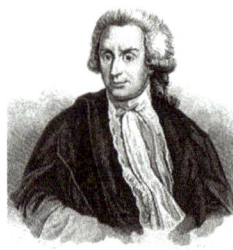

Luigi Galvani and Lucia Galeazzi conduct an experiment on the effect of electricity on a frog

Luigi Galvani
(1737–1798)

Galvani's experiments on how electric "fluids" penetrate animal bodies continued for more than 11 years. The effect was also manifested when a conductor was attached only to a nerve or only to a muscle. Experimenters tried to induce different kinds of electricity, replacing the artificial electricity from the electroforming machine and Leyden jars with natural lightning electricity by connecting a frog's foot with a lightning conductor. During thunderstorms, Galvani and his assistants observed foot contractions during lightning discharges and the passage of clouds. In these experiments, prototypes of future electrotherapy were born.

In broad strokes, Galvani skeched a picture of possible electromedicine methods, revealing the prospects of using electricity for treatment. A hypothesis about the causes of aging is expressed as follows: "...diseases affect especially old people because masses of spoiled animal electricity should accumulate more abundantly in them... ." In those days, electricity was considered a special liquid with a characteristic taste and smell. The whole world was permeated with electricity; in every frog's leg, in every living organ, weak galvanic currents flowed, causing astounding physiological effects. It seemed more than obvious that the brain extracts electric fluid from the blood and the lungs absorb electricity from the atmosphere (it is not for nothing that one can breathe so easily in thunderstorms). The thin electrical fluid, indistinguishable under any microscope, spreads along the nerves, nourishes all the members, and ensures the functioning of all the senses. If one learns how to open and shut off electricity to replace "rotten" electricity with fresh electricity, medicine will make a great leap. Galvani's experiments seemed to convincingly support such a simplified scheme. The main question was where to get fresh electricity.

The market for bioactive supplements of "fresh" electricity developed immediately. In those days, natural discharges of electric fish were highly valued; the price of a numbing eel discharge ranged anywhere from two shillings to 12 shillings 6 pence. In any case, this route was unsuitable for most people; it was a painful hassle to go to patients with electric eels in a fishbowl suitcase. This is why the prototype of electric batteries and accumulators, the Volta pole, an artificial analog of the electric organ of the eel, was so

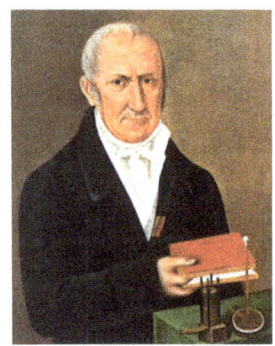

Alessandro Volta
(1745–1827)

enthusiastically received. Just as some optimists have recently considered antioxidants a radical means of prolonging life, at the turn of the 19th century, the scientific world was excited by the idea of reviving the dead with electricity; after all, the severed immobile legs of frogs began to contract under the action of the life-giving flow of electricity. Struck by this prospect, Napoleon generously rewarded Alessandro Volta after watching a demonstration of his experiments; a medal was struck in his honor and a prize of 80,000 ecus was instituted. All the leading scientific societies wanted Volta in their ranks, and the best universities in Europe were willing to give him prominent faculty positions. Volta was later promoted to the title of count and was appointed a member of the Senate of the Kingdom of Italy. Volta's success stimulated the development of various electrotherapy methods in the 19th and 20th centuries, and electrotherapy became the most popular physiotherapy mode.

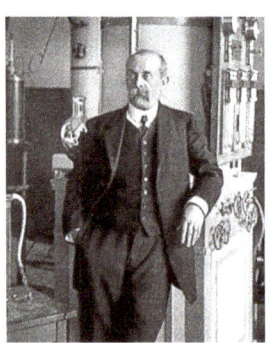

Jacques Arsène
d'Arsonval (1851–1940)

The effect of alternating electric currents is associated with the name of Jacques-Arsène d'Arsonval, French biophysicist and physiologist, a member of the French Academy of Sciences. In 1891, d'Arsonval drew attention of the scientific community to the ability of high-frequency currents to pass through the animal organism without causing tissue irritation while having different physiological effects depending on the application and nature of these currents.

In modern physiotherapy, direct electric current is "embodied" in the method of transdermal drug delivery (Iontophoresis) and various versions of galvanization, pulsed direct current — in the electroporation method, alternating current — in many skin exposure technologies, among the most popular of which are darsonvalization and radiofrequency diathermy.

Electricity, in its various manifestations, has an enormous influence on our lives. For example, being "incorporeal", electromagnetic waves can penetrate and propagate into tissues. **It should be emphasized that waves transfer energy but do not move matter.** The energy can be transformed into heat (which happens in many variants of electrotherapy), which is the main non-specific acting factor. Alternatively, it selectively affects a specific "target" (as is the case in phototherapy methods), putting it into an active state and thus triggering a chain of events. "Realization" of electromagnetic waves inside the organism will depend on the physical parameters of the waves themselves as well as on the physical and chemical characteristics and the biological features of the environment in which they propagate.

There is reason to believe that, in the 21st century, there will be new methods of electrotherapy related to the influence of electric fields on the behavior of cells. The main advantage of the field as a regulator is coherence (synchrony in time). Here we can draw an analogy with television viewers, who receive the same signals simultaneously and therefore act synchronously, such as by doing morning exercises. Thus, fields can synchronize the behavior of many regulation objects. Besides, fields form spatially organized signals, which, in particular, allow cells to be oriented in a certain way. A study of corneal wound healing when subjected to fields of different magnitudes showed that the cell division axis is regulated by the value of transcorneal potential; namely, the higher this value, the more cells orient the division axis parallel to the electric field lines. Electric fields can also determine the direction of cell movement (electrotaxis) and change the expression of certain genes. Learning to control these phenomena is one of the most urgent tasks of modern regenerative medicine.

There have already been breakthroughs in this direction. As we know, our deoxyribonucleic acid (DNA) contains information about the structure of all cells and tissues. But how do embryonic stem cells know in which direction to differentiate to produce a complete fetus? Research led by Michael Levin has identified specific bioelectrical patterns that signal to embryonic cells what they need to become an eye, fingers, gut, etc. (Levin M. et al., 2017). Moreover, scientists could decipher and reproduce these electrical patterns by influencing

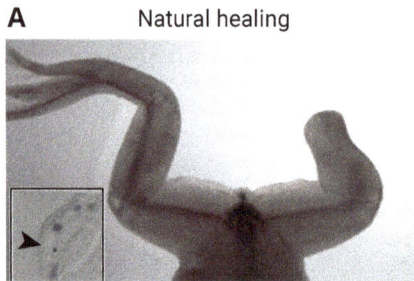 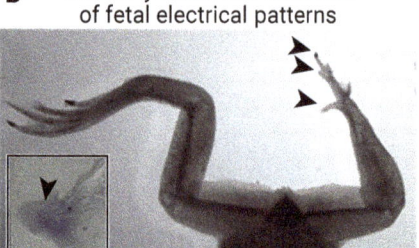

Figure I-2-1. Recovery of the adult frog foot after amputation: A — without external intervention, typically in the form of a simple stump formation; B — exposure of the amputation area to electrical patterns responsible for limb formation in embryos induces growth of a new foot with finger buds (adapted from Levin M. et al., 2017).

special channels and pumps in cell membranes that let ions in and out of the extracellular space. For example, by reading the signal from the cells that would later form the eye and transmitting it to the tail cells of an experimental embryo, the researchers were able to grow a functioning eye on it. After receiving an electric signal that "here must be an eye," a cascade of bioelectric reactions was started, including the fact that the optic nerve found its way to the central nervous system from the tail! In addition, by influencing the electrical patterns responsible for limb formation in embryos, scientists were able to induce the growth in the adult frog of a new paw with toe buds instead of the previously amputated one, as opposed to healing by the standard route by forming a simple stump (**Fig. I-2-1**) (Levin M. et al., 2017). All this opens up amazing possibilities.

2.4. Variety of electrotherapy methods

Table I-2-1 presents the best-known physiotherapeutic and surgical methods based on electrical influence. We will present them all to demonstrate the whole picture of electrotherapy possibilities, as well as to emphasize some principal differences among the familiar methods.

As in pharmacology, in most cases, the stimulating or destructive effect of physical factors depends on the "dose" of exposure;

Table I-2-1. Methods based on electrical and magnetic influences

MAIN ACTIVE FACTOR	PHYSIOTHERAPEUTIC METHOD	
	STIMULATION	DESTRUCTION
The electrodes are a source of current and always touch the skin		
Low-intensity direct electric current	• Galvanization • Drug electrophoresis (Iontophoresis)	• Disincrustation
Low-frequency and low-intensity pulsed direct current	• **Microcurrent therapy** • Dyadinamic therapy • Diadynamophoresis • Electrostimulation • Transcutaneous electroneurostimulation (TENS) therapy, dynamic electroneurostimulation (DENS) therapy • Electrolypolysis	—
High-intensity pulsed direct current	—	• Electroporation
High-frequency (MHz) alternating current	• Radiofrequency (RF) lifting (non-ablative) • RF diathermy	• RF liposuction • RF lipolysis • Non-invasive RF diathermy and electroporation of fat tissue • Electrosurgery • Electroepilation
Low-frequency (kHz and below) alternating current	• Amplipulse therapy (myostimulation) • Ridolysis therapy • Interferential therapy • Fluctuorization therapy	—
There is no electrical contact with the skin, the currents in the tissues arise as a result of exposure to an alternating electric field		
Magnetic field (pulsed)	• Magnetotherapy • Inductotherm therapy • Ultra-high frequency (UHF) inductothermy therapy	—
High-frequency electromagnetic field	• UHF therapy • Decimeter wave (DMW) therapy • Centimeter wave (CMW) therapy	• Radiowave surgery • Microwave thermolysis of sweat glands

the higher it is, the greater the destructive power. In this regard, electrotherapy methods are divided into:
1. Stimulating (**electrotherapeutic**)
2. Destructive (**electrodestructive**)

Many of these methods have found applications in skincare and aesthetic medicine with the aim of solving various cosmetic problems. The **Table I-2-1** shows the classical names adopted in physiotherapy. However, it must be said that, in the aesthetic market, well-known methods often get other names — more "beautiful" and marketing-oriented — which creates a false impression of "revolutionary" hardware technology. Often innovations affect only engineering solutions (ease of use, increased safety) and the external side (attractive design) of the device. As for the principle of action, on closer examination, it turns out that the technology has been known for a long time and has been used in physiotherapy for years. In fact, there is nothing wrong with it — it is even a plus when the technology is labeled "time-tested".

Chapter 3
Microcurrent therapy

Microcurrent therapy relies on modulated pulsed direct currents of very low intensity (in the microampere range, 1 μA = 1/1000000 A) and low density with different frequency characteristics for medical and aesthetic purposes.

3.1. Principle of microcurrent action

It is assumed that the therapeutic effect of microcurrent therapy is based on the **stimulation of potential-dependent ion channels of the cells**.

The cell membrane maintains the constancy of its contents while actively "communicating" with the extracellular environment. Such communication occurs among other mechanisms through ion channels, which are specialized proteins integrated into the membrane and forming channels (pores) for ions to move from outside into the cell and vice versa. a difference in the ion concentration on different sides of the cell membrane results in an electrical voltage; this difference in charge is called the **membrane potential** (**Fig. I-3-1**). By moving ions, and with them the charge, various physicochemical processes in the cell are triggered, and vice versa: various physicochemical processes in the cell can lead to the movement of ions. Essentially, ion channels provide control signals to the cell that "tell" the cell how to function. An example of the extent to which electrical signals affect cells and the body is the work of Michael Levin, which we discussed above (see Part I, section 2.1).

There are different types of channels through which ions are transported. **Potential-dependent ion channels open and close in response to changes in membrane potential.**

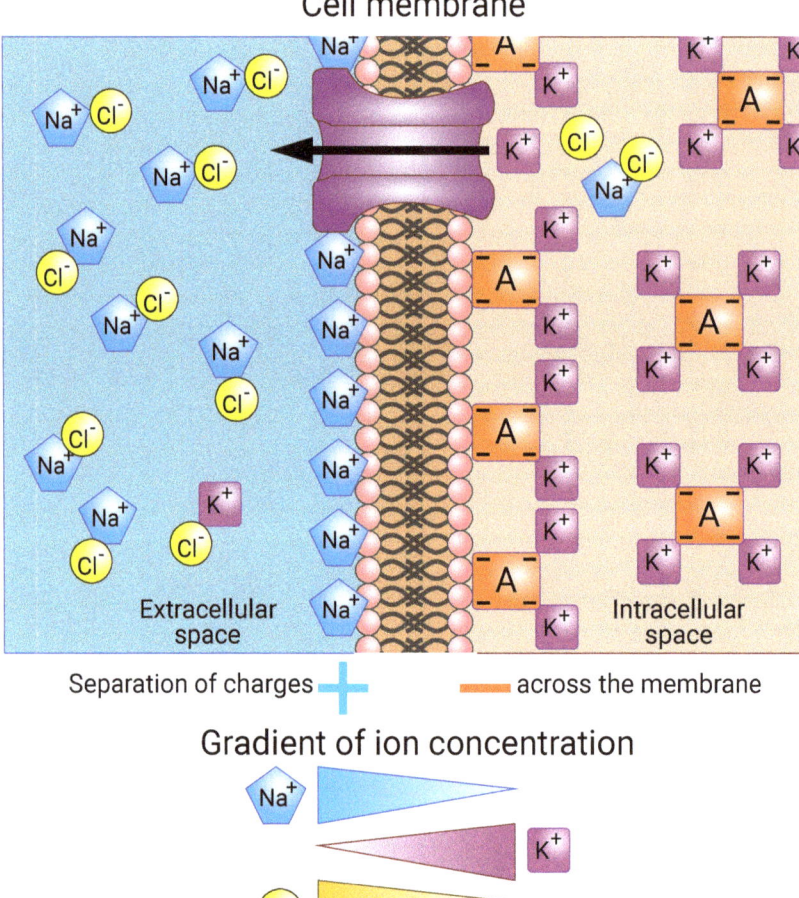

Figure I-3-1. Membrane potential

Under the influence of microcurrent, a redistribution of sodium and potassium ions occurs, leading to a change in the membrane potential. Such polarity "reverse" lasts about 1–2 milliseconds for epithelial cells and 3–5 milliseconds for skeletal muscle cells. At this time, divalent cations enter the cell. These include **calcium** — a powerful physiological signal that triggers a cascade of intracellular reactions, including an increase in the adenosine triphosphate (ATP) level, and provides the cell with energy for metabolic processes (Cheng N. et al., 1982).

Just as mild stresses trigger in the body a chain of reparative processes accompanied by the synthesis of stress HSPs, mild "pricks" of a cell with microcurrent awaken its functional activity. Thus, microcurrent therapy is a gentle method that normalizes and stimulates the work of cells and tissues in general.

The following chain of events is assumed to explain the cell stimulation by microcurrent:

Microcurrent
↓
Cell membrane potential alterations
↓
Opening of ion channels (including Ca^{2+} channels)
↓
Ca^{2+} enters the cells rapidly on a concentration gradient
↓
Increase in the intercellular Ca^{2+} concentration
↓
Activation of Ca^{2+}-dependent enzymes
↓
Increased synthesis of ATP (energy necessary for further intracellular metabolic processes)
↓
Synthesis of proteins, lipids, DNA, and other important biomolecules (due to the activation of nutritional substance delivery into the cell)
↓
Acceleration of tissue differentiation and regeneration

3.2. Microcurrent therapy parameters

It is generally believed that, to achieve the effects outlined above, a microcurrent should have the following characteristics (Bakhovets N.V., 2019a):
- Electric current: up to 600 µA
- Pulse duration: 0.1–1500 ms
- Pulse frequency: 0.1–500 Hz
- Pulse shape: rectangular, triangular, trapezoidal, sinusoidal

Why are such parameters considered optimal? The current (at given frequencies) should not exceed a certain threshold value at which in one period the cell potential has time to change the sign to the opposite one.

The maximal frequency of electrical pulses under the action of which ion channels are opened should not exceed 350–500 Hz for skin cells, 100–330 Hz for muscle cells, and 3–10 Hz for peripheral neurons. If these thresholds are surpassed, the electrical pulses that excite the cell will be delivered faster than the recharge rate of the cell membrane, which will reduce the effectiveness of the action. Nerves and muscles will simply not perceive them as stimuli.

On the other hand, the frequency should not be too low because, in such a case, the number of membrane recharges, and therefore the number of useful substances introduced into the cell and excreted metabolic products, will be lower in a fixed time allocated for the procedure.

The threshold current at which the cell membranes are completely recharged varies for different epidermal, dermal, fat, and muscle cells. Approximate calculations give the following recommended current values:
- Granular and spiky layers of the epidermis: 40–80 µA
- Epidermal basal layer: 80–120 µA
- Hypodermis: 100–140 µA
- Muscle cells: up to 330 µA

However, in addition to short-pulse microcurrent (0.1–0.5 ms), some devices generate longer pulses (100–1500 ms) (Bakhovets N.V., 2019a). Manufacturers have stated that using longer unidirectional (so-called monopolar) microcurrent pulses allows delivering bioactive substances into the skin (see Part I, section 3.9), although with significantly lower efficiency than iontophoresis (electrophoresis). Therefore, if it is important to increase the skin's permeability for an active ingredient, it is better to resort to a specialized electro- or sonophoresis (transdermal delivery with ultrasound).

3.3. Effects of microcurrent therapy

Understanding the mechanisms of microcurrent action allows us to conclude that the effects of microcurrent therapy will be due to

the stimulation of natural biochemical processes in cells: namely, the improvement of metabolism — synthesis of ATP, proteins, lipids, and other compounds. At the same time, microcurrent will affect all cell types:
- Keratinocytes and melanocytes to accelerate the renewal of the epidermis
- Sebocytes to normalize sebum production
- Fibroblasts to activate the synthesis of collagen, elastin, and glycosaminoglycans (hyaluronic acid, etc.)
- Muscle cells (including blood and lymphatic vessels) to stimulate their contraction
- Nerve cells to change their excitability

Thus, the stimulation of metabolism is the main effect of microcurrent therapy. However, special attention should also be paid to its impact on muscles. Of course, microcurrent treatment affects muscle (and nerve) cells because they are primarily sensitive to electrical pulses. In this case, current of very low intensity and short duration is used, very similar to those generated by neurons — the so-called subthreshold impact, which in some way can be called physiological.

Under the influence of microcurrent, there is no active contraction of the muscles, in contrast to electromyostimulation (EMS), where a current of several mA (tens or hundreds of times higher) is used. Microcurrent therapy can **restore muscle tonus**, reducing the hypertonus of mimic muscles (smoothing the facial expression lines) or increasing the tonus of atonic muscles (providing the lifting effect).

This gentle action has additional benefits. The alternating compression and relaxation of muscle fibers under the microcurrent influence acts like a pump. When compressed, the blood and lymph capillaries between the muscle fibers close, and when relaxed, the lumen of capillaries opens, and they fill up again. The effect of microcurrent-induced drainage lasts about a day. In contrast to classical massage, microcurrent therapy is recommended even for severely damaged skin, which is almost the only way to combat swelling associated with such skin conditions.

In particular, microcurrent influences the smooth muscle of arterioles themselves, changing the tonus of the vascular wall. Thus, microcirculation improves, edema is quickly resolved, and cell nutrient supply normalizes, which results in faster healing and restoration of the damaged area. As Thomas Sydenham, a 17th-century English physician, said: "Man is as old as his arteries". Microcurrent therapy rejuvenates tissues largely due to the creation of conditions for a more efficient blood vessel function.

Consequently, microcurrent therapy makes it possible to restore the tonus of weakened or damaged muscles rather quickly and effectively by improving microcirculation. This is especially important in rehabilitation, as well as in aesthetic medicine, because it allows for the non-invasive lifting of the face and body with long-lasting results. It turns out that the declared lifting effect (that is, facial tissue lifting) is carried out not only owing to renewal and restoration of collagen fibers of the extracellular matrix of derma (which, of course, is there, but is not as pronounced as in the case of remodeling due to the action of high-energy methods), but also as a result of stimulation of mimic muscles.

Another important benefit of microcurrent therapy is **pain relief**, which is believed to be realized via the production of endogenous analgesics — endomorphin and enkephalin — as well as direct stimulation of inhibitory nerve fibers that do not let in pain pulses. Microcurrent therapy can also have an anti-inflammatory effect: the level of interleukines Il-1 and Il-6, tumor necrosis factor alpha (TNF-α), and substance P was found to decrease in patients with fibromyalgia after microcurrent treatment (McMakin C. et al., 2005).

3.4. Indications

Microcurrent therapy is recommended for:
- Edema, bags under the eyes, lymphostasis: the effect is achieved by improving blood circulation and metabolic activity.
- Aged skin: microcurrent stimulates epidermis renewal (elimination of fine lines and wrinkles, evening of skin color) and activates dermal cells, promoting the dermal extracellular matrix remodeling. In particular, it restores the facial muscle tonus, reducing the appearance of expression lines and providing skin lifting.
- Maintaining skin health.
- Adjunctive treatment of seborrhea and acne (regulation of sebaceous glands), post-acne scars (activation of epidermal and

dermal regeneration), rosacea, and couperosis (normalization of vascular tonus).
- Cellulite: lymphatic drainage effect, normalization of blood circulation.
- Scars and striae: epidermal and dermal regeneration.
- Rehabilitation after plastic surgery.

Microcurrent therapy helps the skin recover quickly after surgical interventions and aesthetic treatments, followed by altered facial muscle tonus and edema, reducing the recovery period. It is recommended to start the microcurrent treatments on the day after the intervention. At the first stage of rehabilitation (Day 1–7), the procedures are carried out to stimulate tissue regeneration, accelerate epithelialization, and perform lymphatic drainage to unload the thoracic lymphatic duct of the cervical and submandibular lymph nodes to relieve postoperative tissue edema. At the second stage of rehabilitation (Day 8–15), the microcurrent procedure is performed to accelerate the removal of postoperative erythema and prevent possible complications (hypo- and hyperpigmentation).

The simplicity of the method, the low number of contraindications, and the high efficiency have contributed to the wide application and great popularity of this method in aesthetic medicine.

3.5. Contraindications

Contraindications for microcurrent therapy:
- Pacemaker
- Insulin pump
- Metal implants
- Cancer
- Pregnancy
- Severe cardiac and pulmonary disorders
- Fever
- Infectious and viral diseases (incl. herpes infection) in the acute stage
- Purulent processes
- Skin sensitivity disorders in the treated area

- Individual intolerance to an electric current
- Epilepsy

3.6. Microcurrent therapy devices

There are many variants of microcurrent therapy devices that can generate microcurrent pulses of different parameters. Their features are described in the instructions for use, and the "special" effects are explained by the marketers.

In general, we can say that there are devices for microcurrent therapy only and devices combining several skincare technologies, including microcurrent. Regardless of which device is used, the principle of its operation is related to the formation of an electrical circuit through the skin, which requires on-skin electrodes and conductive gel, since the *stratum corneum* has a high electrical resistance.

The probes are chosen according to the treated area and aesthetic objectives (**Fig. I-3-2**).

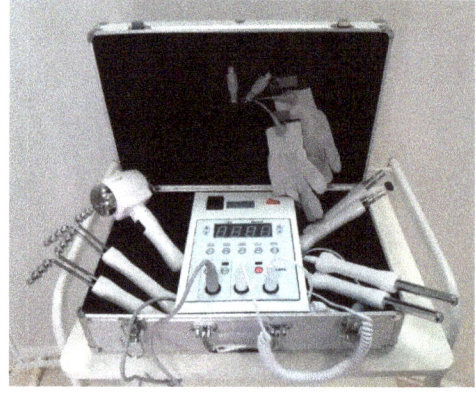

Figure I-3-2. Microcurrent therapy device with different electrodes (example)

- **Probes with metal tips of spherical, conical, etc. shapes** are convenient for local treatment of small non-planar areas on the face, such as around the eyes, but can also be used for large areas on the face and neck. During the procedure, these probes are constantly moved around the treated area.
- **Glove probes** are electrodes made of conductive material that are connected to the microcurrent supply. They are convenient for massage on the face, neck, and body (popular in anti-cellulite programs). Their disadvantage is high gel consumption and the need to treat the gloves after each procedure.

- **Pad probes** are flexible electrodes placed on the treated area. They are usually used with a cosmetic mask. In the monopolar mode, acid and alkali will form under the probe, so the special absorbent hydrophilic cover must be used to avoid chemical irritation of the skin.

In the monopolar mode with prolonged direct current pulses, other probes may be used. In this case, one probe is the active electrode, because the main processes in the skin occur under it. For example, the passage into the skin of substances of the same charge as the active electrode is improved. The second electrode is passive. It is necessary for closing the electric circuit and its contact surface should be at least 1.5–2 times larger than that of the active one. Such an electrode is affixed to the body or hand (Bakhovets N.V., 2019a).

There are microcurrent therapy devices on the market for professional use and home use. However, it is not enough to bring the current to the skin; it is important to perform the procedures correctly, which implies knowledge of physics, skin physiology (for selecting optimal exposure parameters), and even facial anatomy. Therefore, even though using such home devices will have some effect (especially in combination with professional skincare products), the clinical results will be much less significant than those from professional procedures.

For skincare purposes, it is convenient to use a pad covered with a conductive layer on one side (this is the active electrode) and connected to a small-sized pulse generator worn on the wrist (the passive electrode). Under the pad, you can place a special cosmetic mask with active substances, which are selected depending on the skin problem and condition. An example of such a microcurrent device is shown in **Fig. I-3-3**.

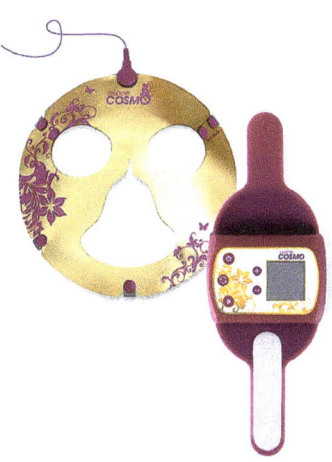

Figure I-3-3. Mask electrode and wrist current generator (DiaDENS Cosmo)

3.7. Microcurrent therapy treatment specifics

There are many variants of treatment protocols, ranging from those recommended by the device manufacturer in the instruction manual depending on its technical capabilities to the author's methods, which are taught at the centers for advanced training. Therefore, we do not consider it correct to give an "abstract" version of such a protocol. To master the possibilities of microcurrent therapy, we recommend appropriate training by qualified practitioners.

The general stages of microcurrent therapy include all standards for any cosmetic procedure:
1. Skin cleansing
2. Toning (moisturizing)
3. Microcurrent treatment
4. Masking with active ingredients (in some cases, it is possible to perform microcurrent therapy directly on the mask if it is current-conductive)
5. Applying sunscreen or other finishing products if necessary

3.8. Transcutaneous electroneurostimulation, dynamic electroneurostimulation

Transcutaneous electroneurostimulation (TENS) and its variant **dynamic electroneurostimulation (DENS)** are forms of microcurrent therapy.

TENS therapy emerged as a method of reflexotherapy intended for pain relief. In 1965, Melzak and Wall proposed the theory of "gate control", positing that nerve impulses caused by a pain stimulus are controlled in the posterior horns of the spinal cord. An attack of pain will occur if the pain stimulus overcomes a certain threshold, which physiologists call "gate control" (gating control). According to this theory, pain signals from other sensory fibers can normally be blocked, resulting in "gate control" and providing analgesia. The gate control theory explains why non-painful stimuli can suppress the responses of the posterior horn neurons that transmit information about painful stimuli to the brain. Based on the provisions of the theory, Melzak and Wall began research on the stimulation of "gate-closing" fibers. The obtained findings led to the emergence of **DENS therapy**, aiming to suppress pain by applying electrical impulses to the skin.

Acupuncture is supposed to be based on a similar mechanism. However, unlike acupuncture, TENS does not affect acupuncture points but the reflexogenic zones of a larger area, such as the area of nerve passage and the areas where pain occurs. Unlike acupuncture, TENS does not cause micro-trauma to the skin.

As a rule, TENS uses pulsed currents with the duration of rectangular bipolar pulses ranging from 0.005 to 0.5 ms and current amplitude up to 50 mA. Stimulation frequency corresponds to two ranges — low-frequency (2–4 Hz) and high-frequency (50–200 Hz).

Repeated skin exposure to low-frequency pulsed current completely inactivates pain impulses from pathological centers. In addition, TENS stimulates the production of endorphins, which are substances that inhibit pain impulses coming through peripheral sensory nerves. Electroneurostimulators are effective against different types of pain. They can be used to treat muscle pain, joint pain, back pain, neck pain, tendonitis (tendon tissue dystrophy), and bursitis (inflammation of the synovial sac). TENS can also be effective in alleviating acute and chronic pain caused by muscle tension.

TENS fundamentally differs from electromyostimulation (EMS) of the neuromuscular system because afferent motor fibers are not irritated, and there is no muscle contraction. The maximum effect is concentrated on the sensitive afferent fibers with high nerve impulse velocity, so the pain impulse from the pathological focus is blocked through the spinal mechanisms.

TENS devices are compact, which means they can be used at home and during trips if there are no contraindications. In addition, many devices are portable, have practically no contraindications, and have no significant side effects.

A disadvantage of TENS is the gradual development of tolerance of somatosensory receptors to stimulation during the procedure. This disadvantage can be mitigated by DENS therapy. The essence of DENS is to affect the skin's reflexogenic zones by short pulses, constantly responding by transforming their shape to changes in skin resistance under the electrodes supplying current, to reduce the adaptation of nerve elements to electrical stimuli. In other words, the pulses constantly change in response to skin reactions (more precisely, its resistance), due to which the receptors practically do not adapt to them. There have been many attempts to use various current modulations and their combinations to lessen adaptation. However, the nervous system remembers these combinations. Therefore, DENS therapy incorporates feedback: changes in impedance values on the skin under the electrode are evaluated and the obtained readings determine the characteristics of a new pulse.

In addition to analgesia occurring directly during the procedure, TENS has a pronounced vasoactive effect, resulting in increased blood circulation in ischemic tissues, metabolic and trophic processes in the exposed area, and deep-lying tissues associated with the skin segments. a series of TENS sessions remove edema and regress inflammation, eliminating the cause of the pain. In addition, the release of endorphins relieves muscle constriction, which improves skin microcirculation.

3.9. What microcurrent therapy should be distinguished from

Within the framework of this book, we directly consider microcurrent therapy, but it is also important to talk briefly about other methods of "small" electrotherapy because a lack of understanding of their principles of action creates the ground for marketing manipulations and/or inadequate expectations from the procedures.

3.9.1. Galvanization

Galvanization uses a **constant electric current of low intensity (up to 50 mA) and low voltage (30–80 V) in non-pulse mode**. It triggers various local and general physiological reactions depending on the body's state, electrode location, and current intensity.

In the skin, mainly in the cathode area, biologically active substances are released. Among these are acetylcholine, histamine, heparin, prostaglandins, endorphins, and blood vessel tone-controlling endothelin and nitric oxide (NO) causing hyperemia. Intensified blood flow stimulates tissue metabolism and promotes skin recovery. Galvanic current also activates sebaceous and sweat glands.

Bioactive substances released in the treated area can diffuse to the underlying tissues and enter the general bloodstream, affecting the entire body. Systemic effects can also be modulated by signals coming to the brain from skin receptors. This explains why galvanic current increases blood supply and the brain's metabolism and has a beneficial effect on the nerve trunks. There is also marked activation of endocrine system functioning, especially of adrenal glands, the pituitary gland, and the thyroid gland. The blood level of free hormones increases, and their tissue consumption is enhanced, contributing to anti-inflammatory treatment.

In general, galvanization has a normalizing impact on the body due to the following **therapeutic effects**:
- Anti-inflammatory
- Analgesic
- Sedative
- Vasoactive
- Anti-edema
- Detoxifying
- Myorelaxant
- Metabolic
- Skin secretion-modulating
- Regenerative

Indications for galvanic treatment:
- Edema
- Post-inflammatory pigmentation disorders
- Decreased muscle tone
- Formation of permanent skin folds
- Seborrhea
- Aged dry skin
- Post-acne scars

- Functional nervous disorders
- Prevention of fatigue
- Hypodynamia

Besides devices for conventional galvanic treatment, there are special **galvanic baths** for feet and hands (current is applied to the hand or foot immersed in water).

It is possible that galvanization effects underlie the effects of "pharaoh's cylinders", which are **copper and zinc cylinders with magnetic fillers**. These cylinders, which were used by the pharaohs and priests of ancient Egypt to enhance vitality and communicate with the gods, are probably the oldest physiotherapeutic devices. Nowadays, by analogy with "pharaoh's cylinders", shungite and nephrite cylinders have been manufactured. Their physiotherapeutic effect is probably based on the electrokinetic phenomena occurring when the cylinders come into contact with the moist skin of the hands.

3.9.2. Iontophoresis

Iontophoresis — from the Greek *iontos* (ion) and *phoresis* (to transfer) — is a transdermal delivery of ionized or charged molecules by supplying the electrodes with the voltage necessary for the movement of charged particles. The classic version of iontophoresis uses a **galvanic (constant) electric current**. Molecules are transported across the *stratum corneum* by electrophoresis and electroosmosis and the electric field can also increase the skin's permeability. These phenomena, directly and indirectly, constitute the active transport of matter due to an applied electric current. The transport is measured in units of chemical flux, commonly $\mu mol/(cm^2 \cdot hour)$.

Iontophoresis uses a weak electric current (0.5 mA/cm^2 or lower). The active electrode has the same polarity as the substance to be delivered. By changing the polarity of the electrodes, it is possible to achieve selective penetration into the skin of certain compounds that, under the influence of the electric field, begin to move through the skin and can eventually enter the systemic bloodstream (**Fig. I-3-4**).

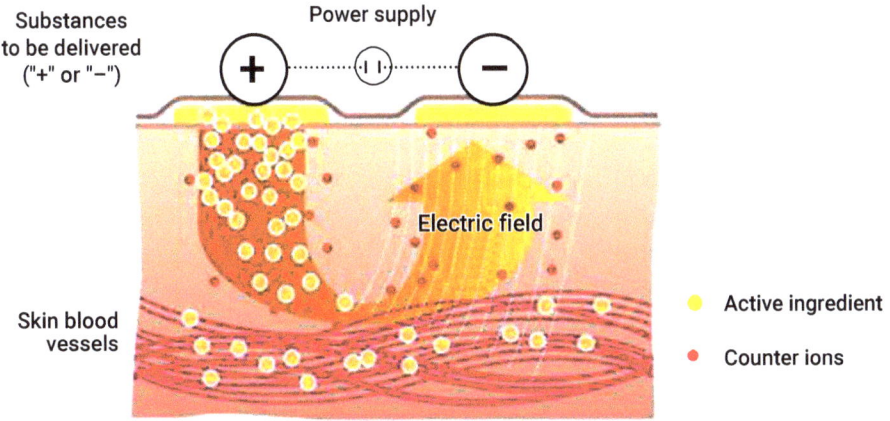

Figure I-3-4. Iontophoresis in skin tissue. Charged molecules are repelled from a similarly charged electrode and penetrate the skin

Iontophoresis increases the permeability of the skin barrier for charged molecules by several times and expands the possibilities of transdermal delivery of drugs into the skin and the body. **Iontophoresis allows predictable delivery because the permeability of the *stratum corneum* is proportional to the current density, which can be easily adjusted.**

As mentioned above, during iontophoresis the same charges are repelled from each other and the electrode with the same charge and diffuse into the skin. Soon after the procedure, the charges are found in the epidermis and dermis, creating the so-called skin depots, from which they slowly enter the body due to the lymph and blood flow. The excretion of substances from the dermal depot takes 3–20 days. This is more convenient than oral medication administration as the patient is not preoccupied with thinking about when to take the drug.

At pH 5.5, the skin surface is negatively charged and acts as a membrane that is selectively permeable to positively charged cations. This contributes significantly to the movement of cations during anodic Iontophoresis. Anodic iontophoresis also involves the convection movement of the solvent, which occurs in response to the movement of counterions. This process is called electroosmosis because water moves with the ions as a part of their hydrate shells. Due to

electroosmosis, the movement of neutral substances and positively charged ions occurs.

As early as 1940, Abramson and Gorin derived a formula to compare iontophoretic current with electric mobility, electroosmosis, and simple diffusion. Particle flux (J_{iontos}) in iontophoresis can be represented as a sum of the following fluxes: $J_{electric}$ (particle flow due to an electric current); $J_{passive}$ (particle flow due to their passive passage through the skin); $J_{convective}$ (particle flow due to convective transport because of electroosmosis):

$$J_{iontos} = J_{electric} + J_{passive} + J_{convective}$$

Penetration of substances through the intact *stratum corneum* can occur simultaneously in several ways:
1. **Intercellular:** between corneocytes
2. **Transcellular:** through corneocytes
3. **Transfollicular:** through hair follicles, ducts of external secretion glands

Ions and hydrophilic substances pass mainly through natural shunts in the *stratum corneum*, represented by the ducts of sweat glands, the lumen of which is filled with aqueous secretion. The penetration of hydrophilic substances through the intercellular spaces is severely limited because they are filled with lipid substances (giving rise to the so-called lipid barrier). However, if the *stratum corneum* is well moisturized before the procedure, the diffusion of hydrophilic substances will increase.

Iontophoresis has experimental, therapeutic, and diagnostic applications. It is currently used for the transdermal delivery of many drugs with low permeability (for example, high-molecular-weight electrolytes such as proteins, peptides, and oligonucleotides, which are usually administered to the body by the parenteral route). For Iontophoresis, a current of low strength is used so that patients experience little or no discomfort during the procedure.

There have been studies of transdermal delivery by short-pulse current instead of constant (galvanic) current. However, the efficacy of this treatment is lower than that attainable with iontophoresis.

3.9.3. Desincrustation

Desincrustation (synonym: electro peeling) is a galvanic treatment with an alkaline solution to clean the skin. Hydrophobic deposits on the skin consisting of sebum, microbiome metabolites, pollution, make-up, and skincare product residues are not water-soluble, so it is difficult to remove them. Desincrustation is accomplished through a chemical reaction called "saponification", in which fatty acids of the sebum react with alkalis, resulting in soaps that are easily washed away and removed from the skin.

Desincrustation is recommended for oily skin with excess sebum production. It is often used in areas with increased sebum secretion (forehead, nose, chin) to soften sebaceous plugs (saponification of comedones). In addition, exposure to electric current promotes the removal of sebum from the pores, increases vascular permeability, and enhances cell metabolism.

3.9.4. Diadynamic therapy

Diadynamic therapy uses pulsed direct electric current with a pulse frequency of 50–100 Hz. The method was proposed by the French dentist P. Bernard in 1946, who called these currents **diadynamic** (today, we also call them **Bernard currents**).

Diadynamic currents excite the exteroceptors (skin receptors that perceive irritation), causing a burning sensation and hyperemia under the electrodes.

A characteristic clinical effect of diadynamic therapy is analgesia, which has two mechanisms behind it. The first is the direct inhibitory effect, like nerve block on the pain sensitivity conductors in the treated area. It leads to an increase in the pain sensitivity threshold resulting in a reduction or even termination of afferent pain impulse cascade in the central nervous system (CNS), achieving a certain degree of anesthesia.

The second mechanism (the concept of dominance proposed by A.A. Ukhtomsky in the early 1920s) is the dominant focus of excitation in CNS in response to a high flow of rhythmically coming signals from interoceptors* and proprioceptors** in the treated zone. The dominant signal of the rhythmic stimulation "overrides" the dominant signal of the pain. As a result, the response impulses from the CNS become normalized, breaking a "pain focus–CNS–pain focus" vicious cycle. It also breaks another cycle associated with the first mechanism: "pain focus–muscle contracture–pain focus".

Vegetative nerve fiber stimulation and rhythmic contraction of muscle fibers in the treated area stimulate collateral circulation and normalize the tone of peripheral vessels, improving blood supply and tissue metabolism. The analgesic effect is partly due to reduced edema and compression of nerve trunks.

The effects of diadynamic therapy on the muscles depend on the direction of the impulse currents. If the electrodes are placed along the muscle fibers, there is an increase in muscle tone and contractility, up to tetanic contractions. Conversely, transverse electrode arrangement decreases the tone of smooth and striated muscles. Many therapeutic interventions — ranging from meditation to electrosleep therapy — help us relax and relieve muscle tension. Diadynamic therapy is one of the most effective methods of relaxation.

The impact of diadynamic current actively affects the blood supply to tissues. In the case of transverse arrangement of the electrodes, there is an improvement in the capillary blood flow and a reduction of the tone of spasmed vessels. When the arrangement is longitudinal, blood flow rate increases by 2–3 times. a positive effect of diadynamic therapy on wound healing, reparative tissue regeneration, and inflammatory processes has been established.

---

* Interoceptors are sensitive nerve endings in various tissues and internal organs that monitor the cardiovascular, digestive, reproductive, respiratory, and urinary systems.

** Proprioceptors are mechanosensory neurons located in muscles, tendons, joints, and skin that detect their work (muscle contractions, movement, body position).

3.9.5. Diadynamophoresis

Diadynamic currents can be used for electrophoresis (diadynamophoresis). This method is inferior to iontophoresis regarding the amount of delivered substances but enables their deeper diffusion. Therefore, diadynamophoresis is preferable for treating deeply localized processes characterized by a clinical picture dominated by pain and vegetative vascular disorders.

3.9.6. Electromyostimulation

Electromyostimulation (EMS) is based on applying electric current to excite or intensify the activity of motor nerves innervating skeletal and smooth muscles. The sensitivity of nerve fibers in the skin and skeletal muscles is approximately three times higher for pulsed direct current compared to non-pulsed direct current. When a pulsed current passes through tissues (at the moments of its rapid activation and interruption), the local concentration of ions near cell membranes changes. This triggers appropriate physiological reactions in the cells of excitable tissues (nervous and muscular). By causing motor excitation and contraction of muscles, pulsed electric current reflexively increases blood and lymph circulation and, at the same time, affects the entire complex of metabolic processes in muscles and nerves.

In skincare, EMS is of limited use because high pulse frequencies often cause a prolonged muscle contraction, which is painful for the patient. Microcurrent therapy, devoid of this disadvantage, has found much wider applications.

3.9.7. Electrolypolysis

Electrolypolysis is one of the options for applying pulsed direct or low-frequency alternating currents to fatty tissue. If pulsed currents are used, electrodes are applied to the problem areas. In case of low-frequency alternating currents, thin, long disposable needle electrodes (8–14 needles) are inserted into the subcutaneous fatty tissue. This may cause slight discomfort. The sensation during the procedure is similar to that of myostimulation.

Clinical effects of electrolypolysis:
- Increased fat cell metabolism rate and fat depot reduction
- Temperature increase in the treated area
- Improvement of blood circulation with subsequent restoration of normal conditions of tissue nutrition, stimulation of lymph flow, and ultimate removal of all decay products as a result of increased diuresis
- Increased muscle tone and strengthening of the skin

Cellulite formation begins with local hypertrophy of fat cells to female sex hormones. Therefore, cellulite is localized in the reproductively important areas (abdomen, thighs, buttocks) with the greatest number of adipocytes due to the biological features of women. Fat accumulation in adipocytes is determined by the balance between the fat synthesis/accumulation (lipogenesis) stimulated by α2-receptors and fat breakdown (lipolysis) stimulated by β-receptors. It has been suggested that adipocyte hyperplasia produces lipoproteins inside the cell located along the inner surface of the plasma membrane, which impede the β-receptor response to stimulation and the subsequent release of fat from the cells. Electrolypolysis activates the β-receptor responsible for lipolysis. a greater clinical effect is achieved when electrolypolysis is combined with lymphatic drainage, EMS, microcurrent therapy, and thermal methods.

Chapter 4
Plasma therapy

We would like to touch upon the use of low-energy plasma (so-called **cold plasma**) in modern skincare as a separate section in this book. This method, which can also be attributed to electrotherapy, has gained popularity recently (Sheptiy O.V., Generalova T.V., 2018).

4.1. The nature of plasma

Plasma is a gas that, unlike the stable gases we are accustomed to, is not only composed of neutral molecules but also includes charged particles — free electrons and positive and negative ions (and in some cases it consists only of these charged particles). As a result, such gas conducts electricity. In other words, plasma is a "carrier" of electric energy.

A gas enters the plasma state when a large amount of energy is transferred to it, which can "tear off" electrons from atoms. For this reason, plasma is known as the fourth aggregate state of matter (along with solid, liquid, and gaseous) (**Fig. I-4-1**). The energy required to reach this state depends on the substance, namely the structure of the outer electron shells of its atoms: the more easily an atom gives off an electron, the less energy must be spent on its detachment. Under natural conditions, the main source of such energy is heating, but plasma can also be attained in other ways. The most important feature of plasma is its **quasi-neutrality**. That is, even though plasma contains differently charged particles, the number of positive and negative charge carriers in a unit of its volume is almost the same. Therefore, the total plasma charge is zero. At the same time, plasma retains the main property distinguishing it from stable gases: the ability to interact with the external electromagnetic field and conduct an electric current.

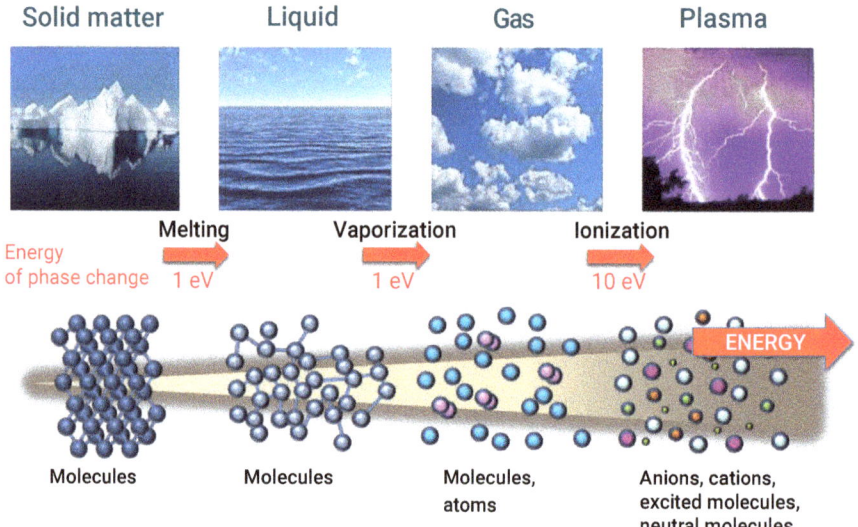

Figure I-4-1. The four aggregate states of matter

- **Solid matter.** In the solid state, matter retains its shape and volume; the molecules that make it up are held together by strong bonds and are arranged in a strictly ordered manner. At sufficiently low temperatures, all substances freeze and become solids.
- **Liquid.** In the liquid state, the substance retains its volume but does not retain its shape. There is an attraction between the molecules that is strong enough to keep them close together but not strong enough to maintain a constant structure.
- **Gas**. Gas molecules interact weakly and move chaotically, due to which gas fills the entire available volume.
- **Plasma.** Plasma is a partially or fully ionized gas that interacts with other charged particles and electromagnetic field.

There are two types of plasma.
- **High-temperature plasma** is in an almost completely ionized state. This type of plasma is present on the Sun, formed in lightning discharges, and under thermonuclear fusion conditions. High-temperature plasma is considered the "classic" fourth aggregate state of matter. Its temperature reaches millions of degrees Celsius.
- **Low-temperature plasma** has a low degree of ionization (up to 1%) and a temperature much lower than the hot plasma

temperature. It is usually obtained when a gas is exposed to a strong electric field, causing ionization of molecules/atoms and directional motion of the generated charged particles. This type of plasma is used in technological production and medicine.

4.2. Biomedical effects of plasma and plasma technology options

Plasma is the source of (Kong M.G. et al., 2009):
- Heat
- Reactive oxygen and nitrogen species (ROS and NO, respectively)
- Electromagnetic radiation — from ultraviolet (UV) to infrared (IR)

The specific effects of interaction with the target tissues will depend on the chemical composition of the applied plasma (nitrogen plasma, argon plasma, helium plasma, air plasma), its dose, flow rate, exposure duration (parameters that can be influenced by device modification), and the characteristics of the tissue itself (Kos S. et al., 2017).

The thermal effects of plasma initially found application in medicine. For example, the high-speed flow of plasma produced by applying a high-frequency electric current to noble gases is a plasma knife used to dissect and remove tissue.

The ability of plasma to heat tissues (although with lower intensity) became the basis for its use in aesthetic medicine (Tiede R. et al., 2014). Plasma methods of skin rejuvenation — plasma skin resurfacing (regeneration), fractional micro plasma thermolysis, etc. — are based on its relatively high-energy effects, as the goal is controlled thermal damage to trigger regenerative processes and tissue regeneration. This principle is the basis of other methods of appliance-based rejuvenation. At the same time, the use of plasma resurfacing technology in low-energy mode gives a superficial impact akin to light peeling and provides brightening and smoothing of skin tone and fine wrinkles (Foster K.W. et al., 2008). The course consists of three or four procedures at three-week intervals and does not require rehabilitation.

In recent years, the technology of low-temperature (35–40 °C) plasma (so-called **cold plasma**), which yields therapeutic effects without damaging living tissue, has attracted considerable attention. For example, such plasma is used for the coagulation of vessels during surgical and endoscopic procedures (**Fig. I-4-2**).

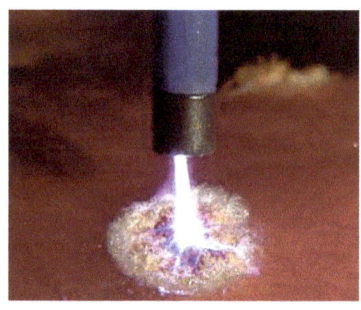

Figure I-4-2. Coagulation of vessels in surgical and endoscopic procedures: argon plasma

The ability of low-temperature plasma to generate free radicals and UV radiation to disinfect human skin and treat wounds is being actively studied (**Fig. I-4-3**). Such exposure makes it possible to kill antibiotic-resistant microorganisms (which is especially important for nosocomial infections) without damaging the skin itself. The antimicrobial activity of plasma has been demonstrated not only in experiments on laboratory animals but also in randomized controlled trials in humans: two-minute treatment of wounds with cold argon plasma caused a significant reduction in the number of both Gram-negative and Gram-positive bacteria in wounds (Isbary G. et al., 2012).

STIMULATION

- Signal transduction (NO)
- Stimulation of angiogenesis (NO)
- Influence on immune cells
- Proliferation of keratinocytes
- Relaxation of smooth muscle fibers (NO)
- Antimicrobial effect (H_2O_2)

Skin regeneration improvement
Skin immunity modulation

SUPPRESSION

- Damage to the cell wall (ROS)
- Oxidative damage to DNA and proteins (ROS)
- Oxidation of lipids in the lipid structure of the *stratum corneum* and increase of the skin permeability
- Suppression of cellular respiration

Infected wound treatment
Transdermal delivery of substances

Figure I-4-3. Biological effects of reactive oxygen and nitrogen species (ROS and NO, respectively)

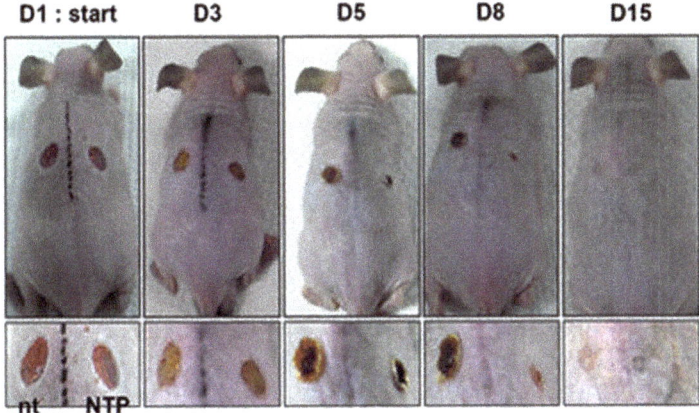

Figure I-4-4. The wound on the left healed naturally, and the wound on the right was treated with cold plasma three times a day for five minutes for two weeks (adapted from Choi J.H. et al., 2017)

It has also been demonstrated that treating wounds with cold low-temperature plasma accelerates their healing (Lee O.J. et al., 2016). Such plasma stimulates keratinocyte proliferation and differentiation due to the activation of the β-catenin-signaling pathway and inhibition of E-cadherin, which is responsible for contact inhibition of cell growth. In mice whose wounds were treated with low-temperature plasma, almost complete recovery of the epidermis and muscle tissue, as well as a high density of collagen fibers, were observed after 15 days, while these processes were much slower in wounds that healed naturally (**Fig. I-4-4**) (Choi J.H. et al., 2017). Available evidence further shows that treatment of fibroblast culture with low-temperature plasma increases the expression of genes responsible for synthesizing collagen type I, fibronectin, and vascular endothelial growth factor (Choi J.H. et al., 2013).

Recent experiments have also revealed that cold plasma causes a temporary decrease in the barrier function of the *stratum corneum* and increases skin permeability to drugs and cosmetics. It is assumed that this effect is due to the rearrangement of lipid bilayers under the influence of plasma and the formation of temporary channels facilitating the passage of various substances (**Fig. I-4-5**) (Shimizu K. et al., 2015). In skincare, such effects are realized, for example, in a device known as "plasma shower". Inside the tip of the "plasma shower"

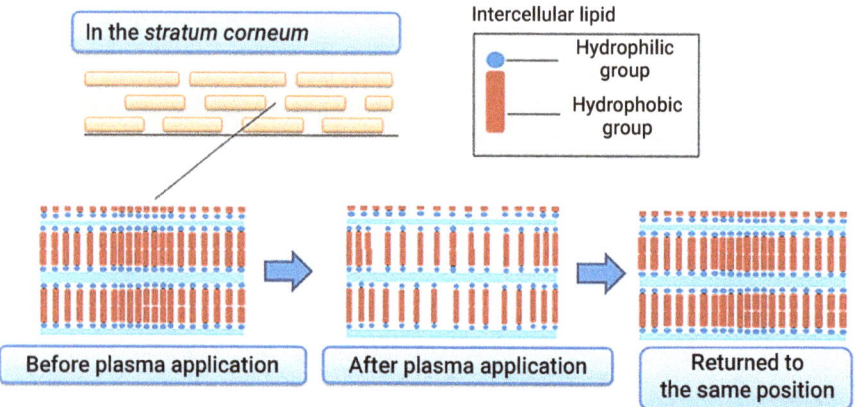

Figure I-4-5. Transient change in lipid bilayer permeability after exposure to cold plasma (adapted from Shimizu K. et al., 2015)

is a set of closely spaced point copper electrodes (**Fig. I-4-6**). The electrodes are separated from the air by a dielectric layer (such as ceramic or quartz glass). When high voltage is applied to the electrodes, a multitude of homonymous charges accumulates on the other side of the glass. An electric field is created between them and the skin surface, and at some point a discharge occurs in the thin air layer between the glass and the skin, which is a flow of ionized gas — plasma (**Fig. I-4-7**). The generated gas discharges between the electrodes and the skin resemble water jets in the shower.

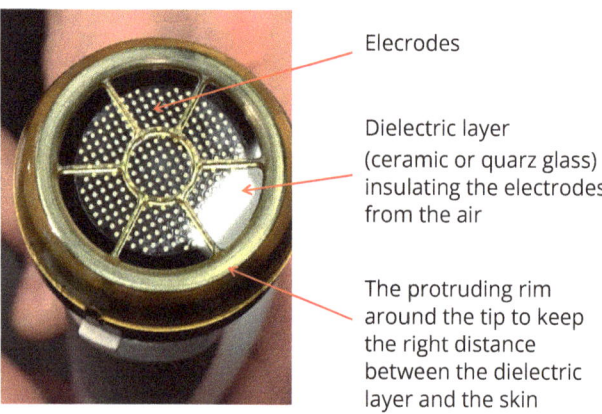

Figure I-4-6. "Plasma shower" tip

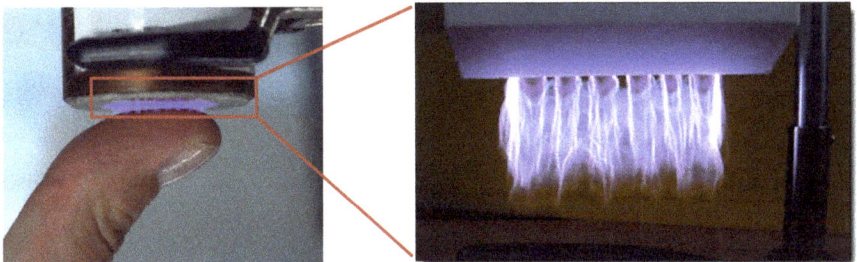

Figure I-4-7. "Plasma shower"

There are many such discharges, and the energy of each is small, but together they can treat a large area non-traumatically and gently. During such treatment, there is surface sterilization, which temporarily increases the permeability of the *stratum corneum* and induces moderate oxidative stress with a biostimulating effect (Arjunan K.P., Clyne A.M., 2011a, 2011b). In addition, plasma affects blood clotting, the immune system, proliferation, and apoptosis of cancer cells (Graves D.B., 2017).

4.3. Indications

Indications for plasma biostimulation ("plasma shower"):
- Inflammation
- Photodamage
- Wounds, chronic ulcers
- Infectious skin lesions (including fungal)
- Transdermal delivery of water-soluble substances
- Preparation of the skin for damaging procedures and tanning
- Rehabilitation after traumatic procedures, sunbathing

Part II

Ultrasound therapy

Chapter 1
The nature of ultrasound

Sound is a physical phenomenon caused by the propagation of mechanical vibrations as elastic waves in a solid, liquid, or gaseous medium. Unlike electromagnetic waves, which can propagate in a vacuum, sound waves do not arise in airless space; they need a "material conductor", a medium of atoms and molecules that will vibrate.

Essentially, sound is the vibration of a medium that is transmitted from a source of mechanical vibration. Examples of sources of sound are our vocal cords, which vibrate as air passes through them, or the strings that a musician plucks. From the source, these vibrations propagate further through the medium, like circles on the water surface, gradually fading away.

1.1. Sound wave generation and propagation in matter

To create an ultrasonic wave, the device first generates an electrical signal, which is repeatedly amplified and sent to the ultrasonic transducer. At the tip of the transducer is a piezoelectric crystal — a dielectric crystal that is able to deform (compress and expand) under the influence of an electrical signal, resulting in a mechanical wave, which is transmitted to the external environment and propagates through it (**Fig. II-1-1**).

When sound waves propagate in a medium, they cause it to deform through successive rarefaction and compression of certain medium regions. The distance between two adjacent regions corresponds to the length of the sound wave. Thus, sound propagation is enabled by the displacement in space and time of the perturbations (displacements of matter particles) occurring in the sound wave.

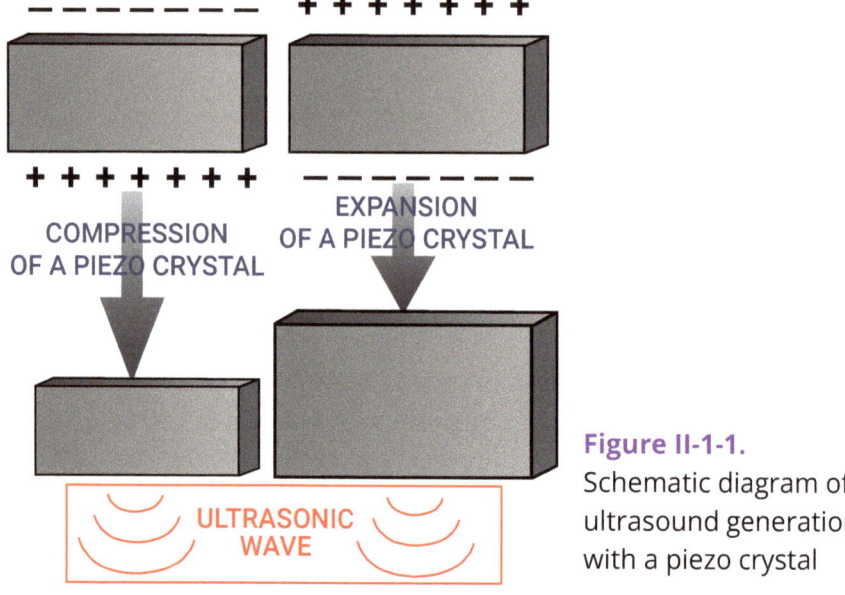

Figure II-1-1. Schematic diagram of ultrasound generation with a piezo crystal

We will now name the main parameters of ultrasound, which determine its interaction with the body.

1.2. Ultrasound parameters determining the interaction with living tissues

1.2.1. Frequency of sound vibrations

Like any wave, sound is characterized by a spectrum of frequencies and amplitude. The frequency of a sound wave is the number of alternations of compression and rarefaction of the medium per unit of time (Hz).

A person is normally aware of airborne vibrations ranging from 16–20 Hz to 15–20 kHz. Sound below the range of human hearing is called **infrasound**; above (up to 1 GHz) — **ultrasound**, from 1 GHz — **hypersound**.

Ultrasound (US) is able to penetrate the skin. The penetration depth depends on its frequency — **the higher the frequency, the worse the penetration**:
- Low-frequency waves (20–45 kHz): 8–14 cm
- Medium-frequency waves (800–1000 kHz): 4–6 cm
- High-frequency waves (1600–3000 kHz): 1–2 cm
- Ultra-high-frequency waves (10 MHz): up to 0.6 cm

1.2.2. Amplitude and intensity

In simplified terms, the amplitude of a sound wave in the audible range is the volume of the sound: the greater the amplitude, the louder the sound.

Just as in the case of electricity, one of the main parameters that will determine the peculiarity of the interaction of ultrasound with the substance will be its intensity. The US intensity is the ratio of its power to the area over which the ultrasonic flow is distributed. This value is measured in Watts per square centimeter (W/cm^2).

The intensity of ultrasound is proportional to the square of its amplitude (loudness). If the amplitude doubles, the intensity quadruples.

For skincare and physiotherapy, ultrasound is used with varying degrees of intensity:
- Very small (up to 0.05 W/cm^2) is used in ultrasonic diagnostics.
- Small (0.05–0.4 W/cm^2) mainly has a stimulating effect.
- Medium (0.5–0.8 W/cm^2) is used for analgesic and anti-inflammatory purposes.
- Large (0.9–1.2 W/cm^2) exhibits a dissolving effect.
- Ultra-high (up to 3 W/cm^2) is used in combination with low-frequency (20–45 kHz) ultrasound for ultrasonic lipolysis.
- More than 10 W/cm^2 causes irreversible changes in tissues.

Ultrasonic vibrations can be delivered in different modes:
- **Continuous** — the source of ultrasonic vibrations constantly works; more intense impact
- **Pulsed** — the source works discretely; oscillations alternate with pauses; less intense exposure

- **Mixed** — prolonged continuous exposure is periodically interrupted by pulse mode oscillations; in fact, it is a variant of the pulse mode

1.2.3. Acoustic impedance

The capacity of the medium to conduct acoustic energy is characterized by its acoustic impedance: the greater the acoustic impedance, the higher the degree of compression and rarefaction of the medium at a given amplitude of vibration of the medium particles. Therefore, the depth of ultrasound penetration will also depend on the properties of the medium.

When ultrasound passes through any medium, it becomes weaker as its amplitude and intensity decrease. This process is called **attenuation**. Three factors cause US attenuation:

1. **Absorption** — ultrasonic energy is absorbed by the medium and is transformed into other types of energy, such as thermal energy
2. **Reflection** — like other waves, when ultrasonic waves fall on the interface between two media with different acoustic properties, they are partially reflected and partially refracted and pass into another medium
3. **Scattering** of ultrasound on inhomogeneities within the medium

As ultrasonic vibrations move further away from the source, the amplitude decreases, as does the energy they carry. This attenuation occurs as the medium in which the sound propagates interacts with the energy passing through it and absorbs some of it. Most of the absorbed energy is converted into heat, whereas a smaller portion causes irreversible structural changes in the transmitting substance. Absorption is the result of friction between particles and its extent is medium-dependent. Absorption also depends on the frequency of sound vibrations: theoretically, absorption is proportional to the square of the frequency. In addition, in the propagation of sound waves, as well as electromagnetic waves, diffraction and interference are possible.

As a rule, the speed of sound in gases is lower than in liquids and is lower in liquids than in solids, mainly due to the decreasing compressibility of substances in these different aggregate states. **The denser the medium, the faster it conducts sound.** On average, under ideal conditions, the speed of sound is:

- In the air: 340–344 m/s
- In water: 1497 m/s
- In glycerol: 1930 m/s
- In bones: approximately 3500–4000 m/s (depending on bone mineral density)

The average speed of US propagation in human soft tissues is 1540 m/s. This is the speed that is preset in most ultrasound diagnostic devices.

Ultrasound is best absorbed by cartilage and bone tissues. When the sound wave passes from blood to cartilage and tendons, the attenuation coefficient and sound propagation velocity increase. This is thought to be caused by collagen (fibrillar proteins).

Adipose tissue and other tissues containing a lot of fluid are the worst at absorbing ultrasound. Accordingly, the absorption of ultrasonic waves by tissues decreases with edema and increases with the formation of scars. Fatty tissue is the most significant living barrier to ultrasound waves.

Energy absorption increases at the boundary between different tissues. To reduce these losses as well as the reflection and refraction coefficient, special contact gels are used in ultrasound-based procedures.

Chapter 2
Ultrasound action on the body and skin

Ultrasound therapy uses ultrahigh-frequency sound waves in the 500–3000 kHz range for therapeutic and prophylactic purposes.

The action of ultrasound on the body is underpinned by five main mechanisms, as described briefly below.

2.1. Mechanical impact

The mechanical impact is based on alternating acoustic pressure, causing alternating compression and stretching. This mechanism is considered primary, and all other effects are secondary.

Ultrasound-induced micro-vibration in tissues changes microcirculation, reduces the viscosity of cell cytoplasm, and breaks weak intermolecular bonds, affecting the dense fibrous scar tissue, which is always pronounced in cellulite stage 2–4. Under the influence of ultrasound, there is depolymerization of hyaluronic acid and chondroitin, which increases the hydration of the dermal layer. Ultrasound massage also stimulates the release of histamine-like substances.

The most radical use of the mechanical impact is ultrasonic lithotripsy, which crushes kidney and gallbladder stones with focused acoustic exposure.

Applications:
- Scars (dermatology and aesthetic medicine)
- Edema (traumatology, surgery, dermatology)
- Hematomas (traumatology)

- Fat deposits (ultrasonic liposuction and cellulite aesthetic treatment)
- Stones in the kidney and gallbladder (lithotripsy in nephrology and hepatology)

2.2. Physicochemical impact

This important cavitation factor manifests through changes in physical, chemical, and biochemical processes.

What is **cavitation**? When ultrasound propagates in a fluid medium, a variable pressure is generated. At the same time, negative pressure can lead to the formation of cavities at the point of rarefaction (cavitation) called cavitation bubbles. They are usually formed in a liquid in the presence of tiny air bubbles, the nucleating centers of cavitation. Liquid and air vapors arise in the cavity. New surfaces form in the cavitation bubbles. As a result of high surface tension, electric charges appear on these surfaces, contributing to the generation of ions in the liquid. When water molecules are split into H^+ and OH^-, hydrogen peroxide is formed, which may lead to the generation of free radicals and biologically active substances, stimulating redox processes. Bubble collapse is accompanied by energy release and temperature increase.

The higher the US frequency, the smaller the size of cavitation bubbles. Low-frequency ultrasound (20 kHz) triggers the formation of cavitation bubbles of 150–300 μm diameter, and high-frequency waves (3 MHz) of about 1–2 μm.

Applications:
- Sonophoresis
- Ultrasonic lipolysis (aesthetic medicine)
- Ultrasonic peeling (skincare)
- Lithotripsy (nephrology, hepatology)
- Ultrasonic teeth cleaning (dentistry)
- Ultrasonic scalpels with the effect of tissue coagulation and bloodless dissection (5–2000 W/cm^2; surgery)

2.3. Thermal effect

The thermal effect is due to the transformation of the mechanical energy of ultrasonic waves into heat. Heating can lead to changes in enzyme activity and blood flow. The thermal effect depends on the absorption of ultrasound by tissues and is not very pronounced, because the heat is removed by circulating blood. Therefore, it is advisable to apply ultrasound in a pulse flow mode, in which the intensity of the ultrasonic wave increases, and the thermal effect will be negligible due to the heat removal by the circulating blood. For skincare practitioners, it is important to note that, owing to some peculiarities of ultrasound, the greatest heating during irradiation of tissues registers on the surface of the bone, which may cause pain, especially in a thin layer of soft tissue. Moreover, unlike radiofrequency diathermy, ultrasound causes a significant temperature increase in the bone without heating the skin.

Ultrasound of 4 W/cm^2 for 20 s leads to an increase in the local tissue temperature by 5–6 °C.

In high-intensity focused ultrasound (HIFU) technology, a special design of the transducer of ultrasonic vibrations makes it possible to concentrate energy in a very small volume with a minimal impact on the surrounding tissue. Ultrasonic waves at the focus cause molecules to vibrate, whereby the resulting friction generates thermal energy and heats soft tissue to a temperature of 60–70 °C. Unlike other high-intensity physical methods, focused ultrasonic waves act selectively, creating a region of thermocoagulation in the beam focus area only, and providing a controlled point denaturation of collagen. The tissues surrounding the area of thermocoagulation remain intact since more than 90% of the energy is released around the beam focus.

Applications:
- Scars (dermatology and aesthetic medicine)
- Skin lifting (aesthetic medicine)
- Contractures in joint injuries (orthopedics, rheumatology)
- Phantom pain after limb amputation, pain in the area of scars and neuromas (neurology)

- To increase the sensitivity of tumors to radiotherapy and chemotherapy, they are treated with focused ultrasound to 43–45 °C for 20–30 minutes (oncology)

2.4. Reflex effects

The reflex action of ultrasound is manifested in analgesic and sedative effects. It is especially evident with segmental influence on certain areas along nerves and vessels. In muscles under the influence of acoustic energy, there is hyperemia, hyperthermia, and an increase in tone. Vascular tone increases under the therapeutic influence. The average dose causes spasms, and high US doses lead to paralysis of the vasomotor nerves. Most patients experience capillary loop dilation after ultrasound therapy and only some have narrowing, which can be considered an individual reaction to ultrasound. Ultrasound has a beneficial effect on the blood supply to the tissues and skin metabolism. Ultrasonic vibrations affect the sympathetic nerve endings of sweat glands and stimulate sweating after the procedure.

Application:
- Muscle spasms (traumatology, neurology, surgery)

2.5. Non-thermal effects

Nonthermal effects of ultrasound include **acoustic currents**, which are unidirectional motions arising from the action of the acoustic field on a liquid medium. The speed of such currents in the liquid in the Doppler scanner beams is 1–14 cm/s, depending on the scanning mode.

Acoustic currents can induce the formation of cavities in tissues where fluid movement is possible. It is assumed that acoustic currents can affect the environment near the membranes, thus accelerating the diffusion of substances through the plasma cell membranes. The fact is that a fixed layer of water molecules exists around cell membranes, which makes it difficult for metabolites to diffuse to the membranes. Acoustic currents seem to erode this layer, thereby accelerating cell metabolism.

Applications:
- Sonophoresis (traumatology, cosmetic dermatology, skincare)
- Acceleration of tissue regeneration and reduction of edema (therapy)

While all ultrasound effects discussed above are used in skincare, in this book we consider low-energy methods such as local ultrasound therapy, ultrasonic peeling, and sonophoresis (ultrasound-assisted transdermal delivery of active substances). Traditional low-energy ultrasound devices generate acoustic waves in the frequency range spanning from 20 kHz to 3 MHz. Devices generating ultrahigh-frequency ultrasound (10 MHz) are also on the market. It is believed that this frequency is better suited for working with the skin because its main effect is realized within a depth comparable with the height of the epidermis and dermis.

Chapter 3
Low-energy ultrasound techniques

3.1. Local ultrasound therapy

Ultrasonic waves used for local treatment are generated by special devices and propagate in a conical beam. The space they permeate is called the **sound field**. Applicators generating lower-frequency vibrations are used to treat the body (where deeper penetration is required), and higher-frequency ones are used on the face.

3.1.1. Biological and clinical effects

Therapeutic ultrasonic vibrations regulate muscle tone, cause reflex dilation of vessels, increase capillary blood supply, and improve the venous outflow of blood. Desensitizing effect of ultrasound has also been noted.

Ultrasonic exposure is used to accelerate wound healing as adjunctive physiotherapy. According to Japanese researchers, the ultrasound-assisted acceleration of chronic wound healing is based on the increased expression of smooth muscle alpha-actin (α-SMA) and transforming growth factor beta (TGF-β) genes (Maeshige N. et al., 2011).

Probably the most significant US effect on the skin is activation of the synthesis of one of the main heat shock proteins (HSPs)* called

---

* HSPs are chaperones — proteins that assist the conformational folding or unfolding of large proteins or macromolecular protein complexes. These "repair proteins" are produced when cells are damaged by various stresses, and their synthesis allows the cell to tolerate stressors regardless of the stressor's nature.

HSP70, which is observed 6–48 hours after exposure to short (1 s) focused ultrasonic pulses. The synthesis of HSP70 has been shown to be significantly higher than the initial level and this effect persisted for four days.

Depolymerization of hyaluronic acid observed under ultrasound exposure is accompanied by the formation of hyaluronic fragments which are important physiological regulators. Moreover, whereas hyaluronic polymers of 100–200 kDa exhibit anti-angiogenic and immunosuppressive effects, the fragments of about 20 kDa have pronounced angiogenic (stimulation of blood vessel growth), immunostimulatory, and proinflammatory properties. Small oligosaccharides stimulate chaperone production and have anti-apoptotic effects. The end products (glucuronic acid and glycosamines) are released from the lysosomes into the cytoplasm to build new hyaluronic acid molecules. Thus, if hyaluronate was previously considered a static molecule ratainig water in the intercellular space, this molecule is now seen as an active modulator of fibroblast activity and angiogenesis. Interestingly, neither the absolute amount of hyaluronic acid nor the size of its polymers decreases significantly with age. However, as we age, the proportion of hyaluronate firmly bound to the protein fibers increases. Interprotein cross-links in the aging dermis impede the approach of enzymes (hyaluronidase) to hyaluronic acid, thereby reducing its metabolic rate. It is possible that ultrasound makes hyaluronic acid more accessible to enzymes, destroying cross-links.

In 2013, Samuels J.A. and colleagues reported on the use of ultrasound applicators for trophic ulcer treatment. In patients with trophic ulcers on whom low-frequency (20–100 kHz) low-energy ultrasound treatment in combination with standard compression therapy was tested, a significant reduction in ulcer size was observed after four weeks of exposure. In contrast, patients not treated with ultrasound had some increase in ulcer size over the same period. The highest therapeutic effect was obtained in the group that received 15-minute sessions of 20 kHz ultrasound. Surprisingly, the group that underwent the same US therapy but the sessions lasted 45 minutes had worse results than the group with the 15-minute duration of exposure. The clinical results were confirmed by experiments on murine fibroblasts: 24 hours after the exposure to low-frequency ultrasound (20 kHz for 15 min) cell metabolism increased by 32%, and their proliferative activity increased by 40% compared with the control.

An ultrasound generator for treating trophic ulcers is made as a compact and light (weighing approx. 100 g) device equipped with two batteries as a source of power supply (**Fig. II-3-1**). Using such a device allows patients to be treated at home without having to go to a doctor, which is especially important for individuals with painful feet. In addition to the ultrasound treatment device for ulcers and wounds, a near-IR spectroscopy-based monitoring system has also been developed. This system assesses changes in the wound in the earliest stages of healing when they are difficult to detect with the naked eye, which helps to optimize the treatment protocol for each patient.

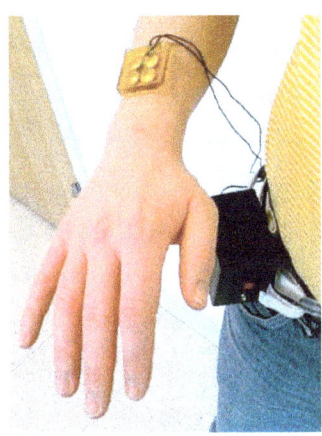

Figure II-3-1. Utrasonic applicator for the trophic ulcer treatment

To enhance the effects of local ultrasound therapy, the use of other ultrasound methods is justified. For example, performing sonophoresis with lidase increases the effectiveness of therapeutic US procedures for cellulite and scars.

A comparison of the effectiveness of ultrasound treatment and ultrasound combined with hyaluronidase involving 42 women showed more pronounced results of the combined therapy (Da Silva C.M., de Mello Pinto M.V., 2013). In the described experiment, the edematous form of cellulite was treated, and the reduction of the subcutaneous fat layer served as an evaluation criterion. Some authors believe that using ultrasound therapy for this type of cellulite and with a similar evaluation criterion is unconvincing (Gulyaev A.A., 2016). The main task of ultrasound is to treat fibrosis; that is, it is advisable to use ultrasound to treat dense and mixed forms of cellulite in stage 2–3 (in the presence of fibrous changes). The same mechanisms dictate the possibility of using ultrasound to reduce the area and severity of scars and striae (Gulyaev A.A., 2016).

Ultrasonic peeling is often combined with ultrasound therapy with the aim of treating age-related changes (Bakhovets N.V., 2019b).

3.1.2. Indications for local ultrasound therapy

The indications for the use of ultrasound therapy in cosmetic dermatology and aesthetic medicine are:
- Cellulite
- Wrinkles
- Scars
- Atopic dermatitis
- Inflammatory skin and muscle diseases
- Trauma
- Trophic ulcers

As in the case of microcurrent therapy, specific exposure protocols are provided by the manufacturers of therapeutic devices and are studied at the advanced training courses.

3.2. Ultrasonic peeling

The corneocyte desquamation is controlled by enzymes (mainly chymotrypsin) that break the bonds (corneodesmosomes) between corneocytes. In turn, the chymotrypsin activity depends on the water level since enzymes can work only in the liquid phase. A decrease in desquamation rate with a constant "pressure" of cells growing from below will lead to the appearance of wrinkles on the skin surface, forming a rough microrelief. One way to break the bonds between the cells and accelerate exfoliation is exposure to intense ultrasonic waves.

3.2.1. Biological and clinical effects

Under the influence of ultrasound, cavitation bubbles arise in the medium applied to the skin. This leads to the destruction of corneodesmosomes and the desquamation of horny scales.

Ultrasound also affects the dermis, especially its dense fibrous structures, "loosening" and accelerating their renewal. The lifting effect observed after the ultrasound procedure is thought to be primarily due to increased dermis hydration, probably as a result of depolymerization of hyaluronic acid and chondroitin sulphate.

3.2.2. Indications

The indications for ultrasonic peeling are:
- Age-related moderate keratosis
- Superficial wrinkles in the cheeks, eye corners, and chin
- Comprehensive care for normal skin

In hyperkeratosis, seborrhea, and inflammatory acne, ultrasonic peeling is not recommended.

3.2.3. Features of ultrasonic peeling

There are many different types of peeling, so what are the advantages of its ultrasonic "version"? One benefit is that, in addition to light "polishing" of the skin from dead horny scales, it also provides a micromassage. Such massage is useful for skin that does not need active cosmetic treatments. Particularly for young skin, ultrasonic peeling can be used for preventive purposes.

Ultrasonic peeling is much gentler than mechanical microdermabrasion. It "works" within the very top layers of the skin. The frequency of the procedure depends on the age and condition of the skin.
- For **young patients with unproblematic skin**, it is sufficient to perform ultrasonic peeling once a month as a preventive monoprocedure.
- For **skin prone to comedones**, ultrasonic peeling (4–8 sessions once every one or two weeks) can be combined with superficial chemical peeling. Such a program is designed for initial seborrhea/acne treatment or maintenance therapy when it is not necessary to mechanically clean the skin. For "old" comedones, ultrasonic peeling can help loosen and soften them to facilitate manual removal later, but it cannot remove them and heal the skin. So, when a patient has already formed acne, it is too late to clean and it is necessary to start acne treatment.
- The accumulation of corneocytes often causes the skin to take on a dull gray hue. Ultrasonic peeling does a good job of superficial exfoliation, and the skin then acquires a pinkish hue and looks fresh and rested. Regarding **stagnant spots, comedones,**

and inflammatory lesions, ultrasonic peeling will not be able to remove these problems and other methods will be needed to solve them.

- In the **older age** group, ultrasonic peeling is usually used when the client does not want to perform chemical peeling and prefers a delicate treatment. In these cases, ultrasonic peeling is recommended for light cleansing and micro-massage. The effect of the massage manifests as a slight pink blush. However, there are certain limitations. Namely, if the patient has couperosis, it is better not to use ultrasound on these areas, as micro-massage can lead to the dilation of blood vessels, which can exacerbate couperosis.

If we analyze the typical target group of clients seeking ultrasonic peeling, these are mostly young people with acne, and people aged over 30–35 years with age-related changes (skin has begun to change its characteristics, the oval face spreads, deepening nasolabial folds). If, at a younger age, the skin was normal and/or had a slight tendency toward oiliness, such skin becomes fine-wrinkled, its general tone gradually decreases, and fine wrinkles appear around the eyes and on the cheeks and neck. This clinical picture is often observed in thin women with normal/combined skin. Vibrating micro-massage improves the blood supply to the skin and stimulates the outflow of metabolites from the intercellular space. After all, even in physiotherapy, low doses of ultrasound exposure are used to regenerate tissues. After ultrasonic peeling, the skin looks better groomed, dullness disappears, and radiance and rosy glow are noted.

Ultrasonic peeling does not require anesthesia. There can be an unpleasant buzzing noise in the patient's ears during the procedure.

The exposure time is 10–15 minutes. The treatment is carried out on a zone-by-zone basis; the sequence of treatment does not matter. The ultrasonic paddle is used to treat the chin, cheeks, forehead, nose, neck, and decolletage area. The transducer blade, tilted at an angle of 40–45°, moves along the course of the pores (**Fig. II-3-2**). Mild hyperemia is common after the procedure, but disappears within 1–2 hours. The manifestation of hyperemia depends on the individual reactivity of the vessels.

There are also ultrasonic peeling devices for home use. These are smaller than the professional ones used in the salon but are also designed for mild cleansing and micro-massage using a gel with appropriate active ingredients. Ultrasonic peeling is usually performed on the face but rarely on the hands.

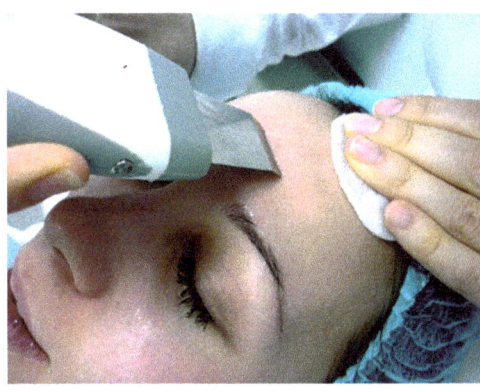

Figure II-3-2. Treatment of the forehead area with the ultrasonic spatula during ultrasonic peeling

Combining superficial and ultrasonic chemical peeling treatments is ideal for those who do not want their skin to scale, as most dead cells will be removed during the procedure. Combining chemical and ultrasonic peeling — as opposed to traditionally using them as separate treatments — can improve the skin appearance much faster, reducing the number of treatments to six at two-week intervals. However, one should not expect a significant evening of the skin microrelief in case of post-acne scarring or significant lightening of pigmentation; this requires more aggressive and deep treatment, and the ultrasonic peeling effect is limited to the *stratum corneum*. The procedure is also recommended as a skin preparation for surgery as it improves the trophic and functional state of the tissues.

3.3. Sonophoresis (phonophoresis)

There are various ways of introducing active substances into the body, but transdermal (or percutaneous) delivery is a special one. The process of transdermal penetration is carried out in several steps.
1. **Penetration** is the ingress of a substance into the *stratum corneum* (this is the rate-determining step since the main barrier structures of the skin are in the *stratum corneum*, and most substances cannot penetrate through this barrier on their own).

2. **Infiltration** is the ingress of a substance from one skin layer to another (the layers are structurally and functionally different, so their affinity to a given substance may vary).
3. **Absorption** is the entry of the substance into the systemic bloodstream.

Routine application of the substance to the skin rarely produces the desired effect because it is blocked by an almost insurmountable barrier created by the *stratum corneum*. The question that arises is how to help the substance overcome this barrier safely and effectively.

Any transdermal system temporarily changes the permeability of the *stratum corneum* without serious damage, which would cause an inflammatory response. It is desirable that the permeability of the *stratum corneum* be restored as quickly as possible to its baseline level after exposure ceases (this is not always possible, however, and in some cases, the barrier remains weakened for some time, during which time special attention should be paid to additional skin protection).

Sonophoresis — synonym: phonophoresis; from Latin *sonus* (sound), Greek *phōnē* (sound, voice), Greek *phoresis* (carrying, transferring) — is a transdermal delivery method based on the use of ultrasound to temporarily increase the permeability of the *stratum corneum*.

According to a biblical legend, the walls of Jericho collapsed under the influence of infrasonic waves. Given the size of the cells, meter-long waves of infrasound are not required to destroy them, as much smaller ultrasound waves will suffice. Studies have shown that ultrasound treatment can lead to an increase in the permeability of the skin barrier. Since the 1950s, high-frequency ultrasound (≥ 700 kHz) has been used for therapeutic purposes; this method is called **high-frequency sonophoresis (HFS)**. The use of low frequencies (20–100 kHz) has become widespread only in the last two decades, and the method is known as **low-frequency sonophoresis (LFS)**.

3.3.1. Basic parameters of sonophoresis

Two characteristics of the ultrasonic wave are most important for sonophoresis: **amplitude** and **frequency**. The amplitude of the ultrasonic wave is proportional to the displacement of the ultrasonic emitter during each half-period of oscillation. The frequency of the ultrasonic wave corresponds to the number of displacements of the transducer tip per second.

According to the frequency, we can distinguish:
- **Low-frequency sonophoresis (LFS)** of 20–100 kHz
- **High-frequency sonophoresis (HFS)** of 0.7–16 MHz (this range includes both therapeutic and high-frequency ultrasound waves, but frequencies within 1–3 MHz are generally used).

Mechanisms of action of ultrasonic waves of **medium frequencies** (100–700 kHz) for transdermal transport are insufficiently studied, so waves of such frequency are not included in any of the above groups.

Other important parameters for sonophoresis are:
- **Duration of the operating cycle** of the ultrasonic transducer (the time period during which ultrasound is emitted)
- **Duration of the procedure**
- **Distance between the ultrasonic transducer and the skin**
- **Composition of the medium** through which the ultrasonic wave is transmitted (the medium between the ultrasonic emitter and the skin can be an aqueous solution or a gel)

Usually, the operating cycle of the ultrasonic transducer is 1:9 (on/off — 0.1 s/0.9 s), 1:1 (on/off — 0.5 s/0.5 s), or there is continuous exposure. As a rule, the pulse mode is used, which makes it possible to reduce the thermal effects of ultrasound exposure because the heat has time to dissipate in the medium.

The distance from the transducer to the skin also varies widely: from direct contact of the transducer with the skin (the gap is zero) to 4 cm. The most common "transducer tip-to-skin" distance is 0.3–1 cm. In the case of HFS, one usually chooses the shortest distance from the transducer to the skin up to the direct contact (the reasons for this will be explained in the discussion of the mechanisms of HFS and LFS action below).

In addition to all the above, the composition and physical and chemical properties of the medium are important for sonophoresis. Viscosity, surface tension, density, acoustic impedance, and the chemical composition of the medium influence the change in skin permeability during sonophoresis. The medium may contain biologically active substances and/or enhancers (substances that increase the permeability of the *stratum corneum*, such as surfactants).

When performing LFS, aqueous solutions are usually used as the medium, while when performing HFS, gels are preferable. In both cases, the medium has an acoustic impedance (a physical property of medium describing how much resistance an ultrasound beam encounters as it passes through it) close to the skin's one, so there is no significant reflection of ultrasonic waves at the border between the medium and the skin.

3.3.2. Mechanisms for increasing the skin permeability

Both HFS and LFS enhance the penetration of various substances through the skin, but their mechanisms of action are different. The mechanisms of increasing skin permeability under the influence of ultrasound are divided into two main groups:
1. Directly related to cavitation
2. Not related or indirectly related to cavitation, namely:
   - Convection (acoustic currents resulting in a reduction of the boundary layer between the skin and the medium)
   - Thermal effects
   - Mechanical effects (exposure to acoustic pressure)
   - Extraction of lipids from intercellular spaces of the *stratum corneum*

The key to understanding the mechanisms of sonophoresis was the discovery of the cavitation process — the formation of cavities (cavitation bubbles) in the liquid filled with the vapor of the liquid itself.

Although not all mechanisms determining the increase in skin permeability during sonophoresis are fully understood, it is generally believed that acoustic cavitation (especially in LFS) plays the leading role. We have already spoken above about cavitation, but we will repeat some key points below. Acoustic cavitation is a process that results in the following events:
1. Microscopic air bubbles in the liquid increase in size or begin to pulsate (oscillate, i.e., expand/compress)
2. New gas bubbles form in the solution or around the crystallization centers
3. Any other type of increase, splitting, or interaction between gas bubbles because of acoustic oscillations in the solution

To understand the mechanisms of sonophoresis associated with cavitation, it is important to consider the size of cavitation bubbles formed at different ultrasound frequencies (Rich K.T. et al., 2014). The radius (**r**) of resonant bubbles is determined by the following equation:

$$r = C / f,$$

where **f** is the ultrasound frequency and **C** is a constant that depends on the properties of the solution in which cavitation occurs.

The higher the US frequency, the smaller the cavitation bubbles. Thus, the radius of resonant air bubbles in the water when exposed to ultrasound of 20 kHz (LFS) is 150 μm, while when exposed to ultrasound of 3 MHz (HFS), the bubble radius is only 1 μm.

The average radius of the cavitation bubbles determines exactly where cavitation will occur. For example, if the radius of the resonant bubbles is larger than the intercellular spaces of the *stratum corneum*, it is unlikely that the cavitation effect will contribute significantly to the increase in its permeability.

In HFS with a frequency within 1–3 MHz, cavitation is the leading mechanism of skin permeability enhancement. The microscopic study conducted by Polat B.E. et al. (2011) demonstrated that cavitation occurs **inside** the *stratum corneum*, in the spaces between corneocytes. This finding suggests that oscillating bubbles directly affect the lipid barrier and change its structure, which leads to increased permeability of the *stratum corneum* (**Fig. II-3-3**).

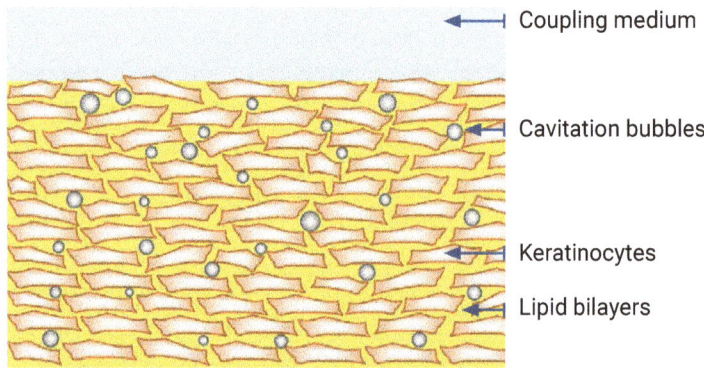

Figure II-3-3. Cavitation bubbles inducing disordering within the *stratum corneum* under HFS (adapted from Polat B.E. et al., 2011)

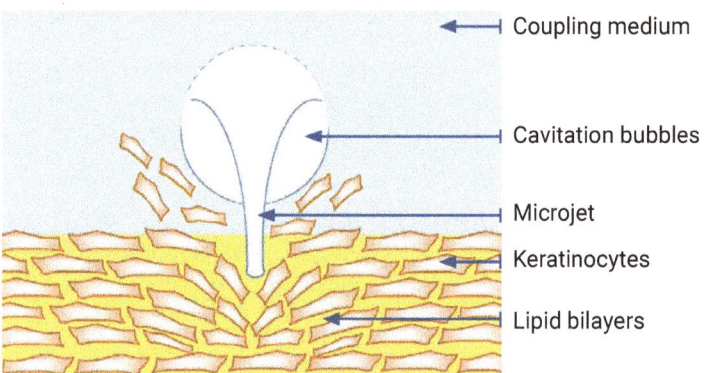

Figure II-3-4. Cavitation bubble asymmetrically collapsing into the *stratum corneum* as a microjet under LFS (adapted from Polat B.E. et al., 2011)

Under the influence of low-frequency ultrasound, much larger cavitation bubbles (with a radius up to 150 μm) are generated, which cannot be formed in *stratum corneum* due to their size, so they are produced in the medium. However, when these bubbles collapse, thin microjets appear (**Fig. II-3-4**) — they "hit" the *stratum corneum* with such force that lipids are "knocked out" from its intercellular spaces, which leads to increased barrier permeability. As was shown experimentally, during exposure to LFS (20 kHz, 15 W/cm^2), up to 30% of the lipids of the *stratum corneum* are released into the medium.

The cavitation in LFS and HFS differs both in localization and in the duration of the skin permeability enhancement.
- **HFS:** the increase in skin permeability during the HFS procedure is more short-lived, and the barrier properties of the *stratum corneum* are quickly restored after the treatment.
- **LFS:** intercellular lipids are washed out from the *stratum corneum*; therefore, more time is required to restore the lipid structures (this explains why low-frequency ultrasound is more suitable for premedication).

The discovery of heterogeneous changes in the skin tissue under the LFS action was of great importance. If the skin is "sounded" with LFS (20 kHz, 15 W/cm^2), a single localized transfer region (LTR) is formed directly under the ultrasonic transducer during exposure (**Fig. II-3-5**). In the LTR, the skin resistance declines 5000 times compared to intact skin. However, if a surfactant such as 1% sodium lauryl sulfate is added to the medium, multiple LTRs form on the skin during LFS exposure, and their combined area can range from 5 to 25% of the skin surface at the exposure site. At high ultrasound frequencies, transdermal delivery occurs more uniformly over the entire surface without LTRs. It is assumed that the collapse of cavitation bubbles with the formation of strong microjets, "hitting" the *stratum corneum*, is the most likely mechanism of LTR formation and increased skin permeability during LFS.

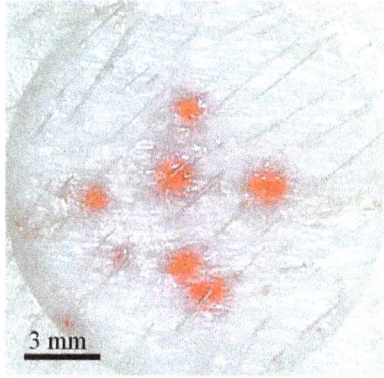

Figure II-3-5. Localized transfer regions (LTRs) formed on the surface of pig skin treated with 20 kHz LFS and a surfactant. LTRs are stained with allura red (adapted from Polat B.E. et al., 2011).

Cavitation should not be considered an isolated process, as it is closely related to other phenomena that may manifest differently

in acoustic cavitation systems. The mechanisms of increase in skin permeability during sonophoresis, unrelated to cavitation, include **skin heating** and **convection**.

Skin tissue is a heterogeneous medium and heats up when ultrasonic waves pass through it. Increased temperature facilitates diffusion of substances in the medium, and, accordingly, substances will pass through the heated skin more easily.

The effect of convection is that, in a liquid medium, the propagation of sound waves of medium to high intensity is accompanied by a unidirectional movement of the medium, known as acoustic current. Acoustic current reduces the boundary layer between the medium and the skin surface, facilitating the entry into the *stratum corneum* of active substances dissolved in the medium. In LFS, as noted, the medium is more fluid; accordingly, the contribution of convection to the overall effect of improving the transdermal delivery of active substances can be significant (see the next section for the synchronized exposure).

3.3.3. Sonophoresis protocols

There are two basic protocols for ultrasonic treatment:
1. As a pretreatment: before the active substance is applied (such exposure is called **premedication**).
2. Simultaneously with the delivery of the active substance dissolved in the medium (**synchronized exposure**).

Synchronized exposure leads to enhanced transport of active substances in two ways:
1. Through structural changes in the *stratum corneum*, leading to an increase in its permeability.
2. Through convection-associated mechanisms, the emergence of which is possible while ultrasound is switched on.

In the case of premedication, amplification occurs only in the first pathway because the substance is applied after the ultrasound is turned off. The synchronized protocol is usually used in HFS studies. Both protocols are found in LFS research, but premedication is used more frequently, including the clinical application of sonophoresis. There are three reasons for this choice of protocol.

First, exposure of a drug or other active substance to ultrasound can lead to the degradation of its molecules or other chemical reactions. As a result, the substance may lose its biological activity or undergo unwanted changes that will produce compounds harmful to humans.

Second, the synchronized protocol requires the ultrasound transducer to be near the person until the substance has fully penetrated the skin, whereas for premedication, a short-term (about 10 s) ultrasound exposure is sufficient.

Third, a much greater increase in skin permeability can be achieved with LFS than with HFS, allowing LFS to be used as premedication to deliver therapeutic doses of drugs without the additional use of the convection mechanism.

3.3.4. Opportunities and limitations

A valuable practical observation regarding sonophoresis as a method of transdermal delivery is the finding that the simultaneous use of sonophoresis and chemical enhancers (primarily surfactants) leads to synergistic action and facilitates transdermal passage. The combined effects of LFS and surfactants dissolved in the medium can be divided into two mechanisms:
1. Surfactants' effect on the ultrasound-associated phenomena
2. The effect of ultrasound on surfactants' penetration, dispersion, and decomposition (cleavage) in the skin

Most of the compounds delivered with HFS are molecules up to 1000 Da in size; only a few trials have been performed to deliver molecules exceeding 1000 Da molecular mass. This delineation suggests that HFS does not change the skin's structure much and can therefore be used mainly to deliver molecules that would penetrate the skin under normal conditions but in smaller amounts.

The fact that HFS does not cause significant changes in the skin structure is beneficial and confirms that the technology is safe and can be widely used in skincare, physical therapy, and sports medicine.

To date, the use of HFS for transdermal delivery has been investigated for more than 90 different drug compounds, and there are many areas of interest in applying therapeutic high-frequency ultrasound for this purpose. The most common types of HFS-administered substances are anti-inflammatory drugs for treating joint and muscle pain and ointments for the local treatment of skin or muscle conditions.

Compared to HFS, LFS has expanded the list of compounds that can be administered through the skin in therapeutic doses. These include various hydrophilic or hydrophobic substances, as well as substances with small (up to 1000 Da) and high (≥ 1000 Da) molecular masses. Therefore, LFS may find wider application than HFS, despite some obstacles to its full-fledged use due to the lack of safety justifications for this method. The use of LFS for transdermal vaccination is by far the most actively developing area of research. Another advantage of LFS transdermal delivery is that its therapeutic efficacy is often as good as that of intramuscular injection, with reduced antigen consumption.

Another promising area of research is the LFS-transdermal administration of drug carriers. Several groups of scientists have recently demonstrated the ability of LFS to transport nanoparticles of 100-nm size through the *stratum corneum* into the viable epidermal and dermal layers (Tawfik M.A. et al., 2020).

Sonophoresis can also be combined with physical therapy treatments such as electroporation, Iontophoresis, and dermabrasion. Synergy between HFS and electroporation has already been demonstrated; the use of HFS alone had no effect on the passage of the fluorescent dye calcein through the *stratum corneum*, but in combination with electroporation, the flow of calcein increased twofold compared to that observed with electroporation alone (Daftardar S. et al., 2019). The combination of LFS with iontophoresis proved to be justified, but this combined method of transdermal delivery was not suitable for all substances: the best result was shown for non-ionized compounds or those over 1000 Da, while skin permeability for ionized molecules remained at the same level as when Iontophoresis was used alone (Daftardar S. et al., 2019).

Part III

LED therapy (Photobiomodulation)

Light is widely used in skin physiotherapy. Depending on what the light source is, there are two basic groups of light technologies:
1. **Lamp** — xenon lamps in intense pulsed light (IPL) devices, light-emission diodes (LED)
2. **Laser** — solid-state, gas, liquid (dye), and semiconductor (laser diode) lasers

We discuss light technology in detail in the *Lasers in Cosmetic Dermatology & Skincare Practice* book. Here, we will focus only on one method, which is known by several names: **LED therapy**, **low-level laser (light) therapy (LLLT)**, and **photobiomodulation**. These terms are synonymous and refer to a specific technology that uses low-level laser radiation in the red and infrared (IR) spectrum to affect the skin.

Unlike electricity and sound, which have no specific target in the medium through which they propagate, light does have such a target — these are atoms and molecules of a substance absorbing electromagnetic radiation of certain wavelengths. Each atom and molecule possesses a specific absorption spectrum — a kind of "identity card", by which we can determine the presence of certain substances in the environment.

The selectivity of light absorption by each molecular target underlies its therapeutic application. When using light to treat the skin, there are three main targets: melanin, hemoglobin, and water. When treating pigmentary and vascular disorders, removing unwanted hair, and rejuvenating the skin, it is these substances that are the acceptors of light energy. They are selectively heated, destroyed (partially or completely), and/or trigger a sequence of processes in the skin that lead to a clinical result.

However, the physical treatment discussed in this section has another target and mechanism of action. Before we get to it, let us briefly discuss the nature of light.

Chapter 1
The nature of light

1.1. Light and its parameters

Light is electromagnetic radiation emitted by heated or excited matter.

In everyday life, we think of light as what we can see with our eyes — radiation in the visible range of the electromagnetic spectrum. However, this is just a very small part of it (**Fig. III-1-1**). The electromagnetic spectrum includes different types of electromagnetic radiation that differ from each other in frequency, wavelength, and energy transfer power. All these parameters will determine their properties and the characteristics of light interaction with biological tissues. Optical (visible) radiation, or light, is electromagnetic radiation with a wavelength ranging from 100 nm (UV range) to 1000 μm (IR range).

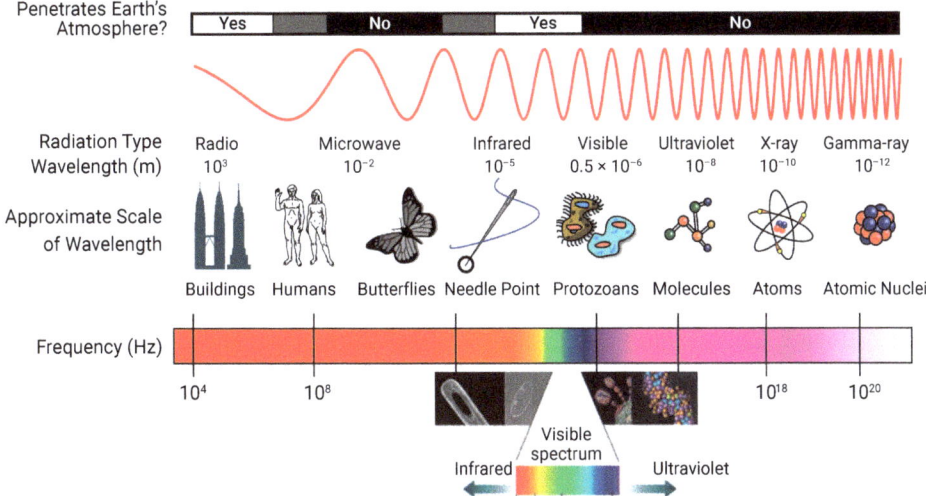

Figure III-1-1. Electromagnetic spectrum

Electromagnetic radiation consists of electromagnetic waves, which are synchronized oscillations of electric and magnetic fields.

Electromagnetic waves, like any other periodically repeating process, are characterized by frequency. The **frequency of electromagnetic waves (ν)** is the number of crests that pass a given point (observer, detector, etc.) per second. For example, a frequency of 1 Hz is equivalent to one oscillation per second, and of 1 megahertz (MHz) is a million oscillations per second.

Another qualitative characteristic, wavelength, is often used when describing wave processes. **Wavelength (λ)** is the distance between two adjacent crests of the wave, which is measured in units of length (nm, mm, etc.) (**Table III-1-1**).

Table III-1-1. Optical spectral bands

TYPE OF RADIATION	WAVELENGTH
Ultraviolet (UV) radiation	**100–400 nm**
Ultraviolet type C (UVC), shortwave	100–280 nm
Ultraviolet type B (UVB), medium-wave	280–315 nm
Ultraviolet type a (UVA), longwave	315–400 nm
Visible (optical) radiation	**400–760 nm**
Purple	400–450 nm
Blue	450–480 nm
Blue	480–510 nm
Green	510–575 nm
Yellow	575–585 nm
Orange	585–620 nm
Red	620–760 nm
Infrared (IR) radiation*	**760 nm – 1000 μm**
Near-IR	760 nm – 3 μm
Mid-IR	3–50 μm
Far-IR	50–1000 μm

* The classification of IR radiation ranges by different regulatory authorities varies. The ranges provided here are given by the International Organization for Standardization (ISO).

Natural sources of light (fire in combustion, sun) and lamps (incandescent, discharge, fluorescent) emit light in all directions, panoramically. There are many different wavelengths in the emitted spectrum, and its characteristics depend on the emitting material. Since light sources vary in chemical composition, their emission spectra will also differ. In addition, their radiation is non-polarized, i.e., oscillations of the electric and magnetic fields of different photons are in different planes. Therefore, even if a light beam comes out from a narrow hole (for example, the lamp is placed in a closed box in which a hole is made), it will diverge. The phenomenon of beam divergence is clearly visible when comparing the light spots on the obstacles located at different distances from the exit hole; the farther the object, the larger the light spot.

Unlike natural and lamp sources, **laser light** is monochromatic (that is, its spectrum contains waves of the same length) and polarized (oscillations of electric and magnetic fields of all photons occur in single perpendicular planes). The laser beam does not diverge when moving away from the source, which ensures its maximum focus. Due to these features, laser radiation allows for a more precise control of the impact on the target. Monochromatic polarized radiation does not exist in nature; producing it requires special light generators called **lasers**.

1.2. Laser devices

Laser is an acronym for **L**ight **A**mplification by **S**timulated **E**mission of **R**adiation.

The starting point for laser development was the work of Albert Einstein. In 1916, he promulgated his famous Theory of Relativity and introduced to the scientific community the concept of induced radiation, which became the basis for the development of lasers. It was preceded by the discovery that, when an electron moves from the upper high-energy level to a lower-energy level, the difference between the energies of these levels is emitted as photons characterized by a certain wavelength, which depends on the energy difference between the electronic levels, i.e., on the characteristics of a particular chemical element.

Einstein suggested that when such a photon hits a medium with many excited structures identical to the "parent" ones, it induces the transition of the quantum system (atom/molecule) from the excited to the stable state. In other words, electrons return to their stable levels, generating a new photon with the same wavelength, energy, and polarization as the primary photon. In turn, the new photon will affect other excited structures similarly, resulting in a chain reaction. That is, there will be light amplification by stimulated emission of radiation (laser). As a result, a weak flux of light in the laser environment is amplified, and not chaotically, but in one given direction. Thus, we can get an "amplified" light flux with completely predictable characteristics.

How exactly does this happen?

1.2.1. How lasers work

A laser is an optical frequency oscillator — a device that converts initial energy (light, electrical, thermal, chemical) into a laser beam.

A laser has three main components: the active (or gain) medium, the energy source, and the resonant cavity (optical resonator). The active medium is a material composed of atoms or molecules which provide the electrons needed to emit photons. The active medium can be a solid, a liquid, or a gas.

When the device is switched off, all quantum systems (atoms, molecules) of its active medium are in a ground state — electrons occupy a stable position on their basic orbitals. When energy is applied, the so-called **pumping** occurs. Laser pumping is the act of energy transfer from an external source into the gain medium. The energy is absorbed in the medium, producing excited states in its atoms. Since this state is extremely unstable, individual atoms can spontaneously return to a ground state (an electron from a higher level will return to the ground one), and the excess energy will be released as a quantum of light (photon). Reflecting from special mirrors (**optical resonators**), it will return to the laser gain medium. Here, the mechanism of stimulated emission is triggered: as mentioned above, such a photon induces the transition of neighbors from an excited state to a stable state with the emission of fully identical photons, while it itself is not absorbed and continues to affect other excited atoms of the medium, as well as newly formed photons (**Fig. III-1-2**).

A. Absorption of energy (light, electrical, thermal, chemical)

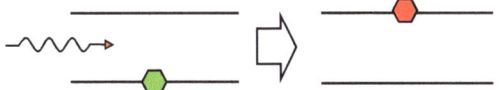

B. Spontaneous emission of radiation

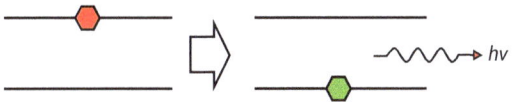

C. Stimulated emission of radiation

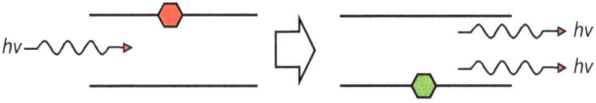

h — Planck's constant, a fundamental universal constant that defines the quantum nature of energy and relates the energy of a photon to its frequency.

Figure III-1-2. Induction of stimulated emission

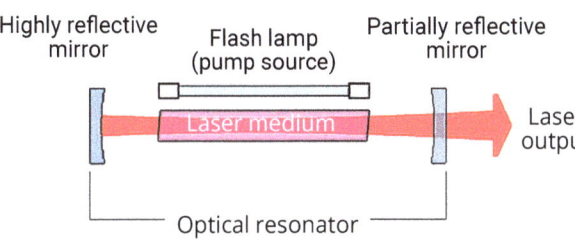

Figure III-1-3. Schematic diagram of a laser device

The laser gain medium is located in the optical resonator with two mirrors on opposite walls facing each other. The rear mirror reflects the entire flux of photons produced, while the other mirror is partially transparent (**Fig. III-1-3**). Through a series of multiple reflections, enough photons accumulate, all of which together "break through" the front mirror. The result is an overall laser beam with fully identical emission characteristics: the greater the number of electrons that return to their ground levels, the more powerful it will be.

In simple terms, unlike the lighting devices we are familiar with — incandescent lamps, flashlights, and even the Sun, which emits all generated photons into the environment — a laser makes it possible to retain and "reproduce" photons (which will all be "cloned"; that is, identical to each other), and then release them in the form of a focused beam. Such "cloning" will be responsible for the unique properties of laser radiation.

1.2.2. Laser types

Laser devices differ in terms of the gain medium in which the stimulated radiation is formed.

- **Solid-state lasers** — the gain medium is a crystal or glass enriched with chromium, erbium, neodymium, or titanium ions. a pulsed lamp or another laser pumps the solid-state laser. These are the most common types of lasers used in dermatology (at least, they were before the advent of laser diodes), e.g., ruby (Rubi, 694 nm), alexandrite (Alex, 732 nm), neodymium-doped yttrium-aluminum-garnet (Nd:YAG, 1064 nm), and erbium-doped yttrium-aluminum-garnet (Er:YAG, 2940 nm) lasers.
- **Liquid lasers** — the gain medium consists of an organic solvent and a dye. The laser is pumped by a pulsed lamp or another laser. Their advantage is that they can be tuned in a wide spectral range. Liquid lasers include dye lasers, such as pulsed dye laser (PDL) that generates radiation with a wavelength of 575–595 nm and is used to treat vascular lesions.
- **Gas lasers** may contain carbon dioxide (CO_2, 10,600 nm), krypton (460–680 nm), argon (488–514 nm), or gas mixtures (they are pumped by electrical discharges). The CO_2 laser is one of the most powerful and most common in medicine.
- **Excimer lasers** are gas lasers with gain compounds that can exist only in an excited state; that is, xenon–chlorine (XeCl, 308 nm), xenon–fluorine (XeF, 351 nm), helium–neon (HeNe, 633 nm), etc.
- **Semiconductor lasers** contain semiconductor crystal like gallium arsenide (GaAs, 820 nm) as a gain medium. The fundamental difference between semiconductor and solid-state laser is that the stimulated emission in the former is formed not by the transition of electrons between levels, but by the transitions between energy bands or subzones of the crystal. Pumping is done by electric current.

The most typical example of a semiconductor laser is a **diode laser**. Although diode lasers were invented almost simultaneously with the first lasers, they were not used in dermatology for a long time. However, the last decade has seen an unequivocal boom in their popularity. There are at least two reasons for this upward trend.

First, semiconductor lasers are characterized by a much higher radiation yield than other types of lasers. In this case, efficiency is the ratio of the power generated by the laser to the power consumed by the laser device to generate it. In other words, it is the ratio of the light energy emitted to the energy expended to produce it. Gas lasers have an efficiency of 1–20% (HeNe — up to 1%, CO_2 — 10–20%), solid-state lasers — 1–6%, and diode lasers — 10–50% (in some designs up to 95%) (Moskvin S.V., 2016). Due to this fact, these lasers can (and do) have a very small gain medium compartment and consume less energy (current strength — tens of mA, voltage — up to 10 V), while "classical" lasers can require thousands of volts. Thus, diode lasers are quite compact and do not require any special conditions for operation.

Second, laser diodes can generate radiation in the 365–9000 nm wavelength range (depending on the crystal material and the presence of impurities in the active medium). It is possible to fine-tune the spectrum and power of radiation (Moskvin S.V., 2016).

In addition to lasers, there are also so-called **light-emitting diodes (LEDs)**, thanks to which LED therapy got its name (although some devices can also operate on laser diodes). Strictly speaking, light-emitting diodes are not the same as laser diodes. While LEDs are also semiconductor-based devices, they use different types of semiconductors — electron-conducting and hole-conducting. When electric current passes between these different semiconductors, incoherent radiation is generated. Although it has a narrower spectrum (usually within a dozen nm) than conventional thermal light sources and makes it possible to obtain specific light, it is still not coherent. In addition, LEDs cannot be operated in pulsed mode, which is the most effective mode of laser exposure as it makes it possible to level out some undesirable biological effects of laser radiation and to increase the accuracy and efficiency of procedures.

Devices based on light-emitting diodes are simple enough to design, quite cheap, and do not require consumables and special maintenance, but they are reliable, which has made them very popular in skincare. At the same time, modern technology allows producing flexible matrices, which makes it possible to develop devices of complex shapes, such as masks and flexible panels (**Fig. III-1-4**). However, their efficiency will be lower than that of laser diodes because precision is crucial for exposure to biological tissues. This is especially true for low-intensity exposure, where we don't just want to destroy the target, but to give it a precise (both in wavelength and energy) stimulus to work.

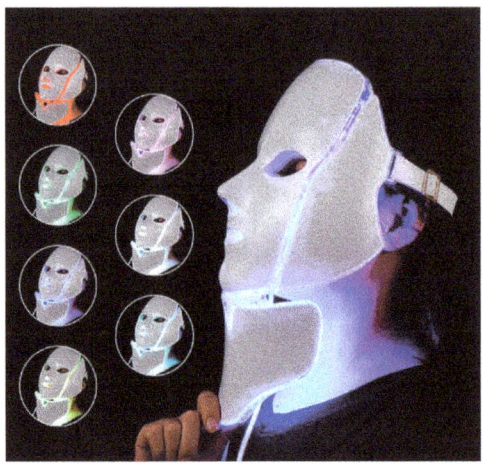

Figure III-1-4. LED face and neck skincare mask

1.3. Basic parameters of laser radiation that determine laser–target interactions

The main physical parameters determining the peculiarities of the action of lasers on biological tissues are:
- Wavelength of the generated radiation
- Energy fluence and power
- Duration and mode of irradiation (pulsed or continuous)
- Light spot size and the ability to focus the energy

1.3.1. Wavelength of the generated radiation

The **wavelength (λ)** of laser radiation is determined by its gain medium and defines the characteristics of absorption of the emitted light by individual skin structures. Each substance (so-called chromophore) has its own absorption spectrum — a curve showing how a given substance absorbs radiation of different wavelengths. Thus, by selecting a certain wavelength depending on the absorption spectrum of the skin chromophores, we can target certain skin structures.

The wavelength also determines the depth of light penetration into the skin: **the longer the wavelength, the deeper the penetration of light radiation into the skin. IR rays** penetrate into the tissue to a depth of up to 7 cm, visible light to 1 cm, and UV rays to 0.5–1.0 mm (**Table III-1-2**, **Fig. III-1-5**). At the same time, the wavelength is inversely proportional to the light energy. This means that short-wavelength radiation has a higher energy than a long-wavelength light beam.

Therefore, if we want to treat some specific skin structures with laser, both the absorption peaks of the target chromophores and the depth of the structures containing them should be considered.

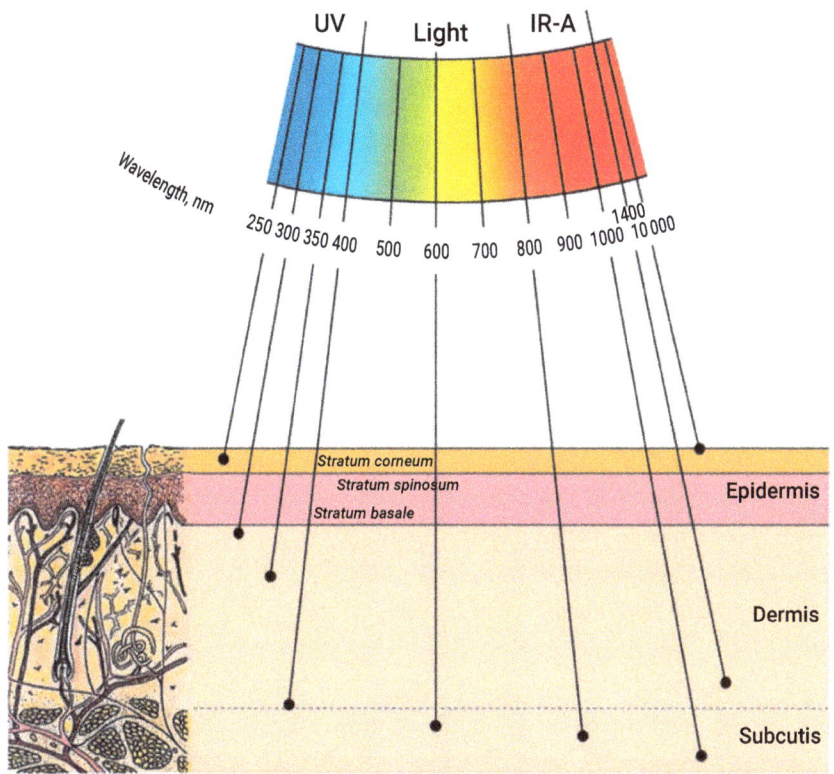

Figure III-1-5. Depth of light penetration as a function of emission wavelength

Table III-1-2. Spectral bands of optical radiation and their depth of penetration into the skin

SPECTRAL BAND	SKIN PENETRATION DEPTH (PHOTONS PENETRATING TO A GIVEN DEPTH, %)
UVC	30 µm (5%)
UVB	30 µm (33%)
UVA	30 µm (50%)
Colored bands: violet to red	1 mm (blue) (50%); 10 mm (red) (60%)
Near-IR	30–40 mm (60%)
Far-IR	

1.3.2. Energy density (fluence) and power

How pronounced the effect on the chromophore will be and what impact it will have on the target structure depends on the **energy (J)** of the laser radiation and its **power (W)**, which characterizes the rate of delivery of this energy. In practice, these parameters are used in terms of **energy density (fluence) (J/cm²)** and **power density (energy flux density) (W/cm²)** per unit area.

It is important to remember that only the absorbed dose has a biological effect because part of the light is reflected by the skin. Note that skin reflects about 60% of IR rays, 40% of visible light, and 10% of UV rays. For UV and visible rays, the reflectivity of unpigmented skin is almost twice as high as that of pigmented skin. In the infrared region, the reflectivity of light skin is about 20% higher.

In terms of radiation power, medical lasers are divided into:
- Low-power lasers: 1–5 mW
- Medium-power lasers: 6–500 mW
- High-power lasers: over 500 mW

Low- and medium-power lasers are counted among **biostimulation lasers**. It is these lasers that we will discuss within the scope of this book. High-power lasers are referred to as photo-destructive lasers and are used for laser resurfacing procedures, fractional photothermolysis, laser removal of neoplasms, etc.

1.3.3. Laser operating mode: pulsed or continuous

Laser light can be delivered to the skin continuously or in pulses. For pulsed mode, the pulse frequency is important. It is measured in pulses per second (Hz). Pulse duration and power are also important. For continuous mode, the average exposure power will be constant, and will be significantly greater than for pulsed mode, in which the power of a single pulse can be high.

1.3.4. Light spot and energy focusing

For skincare and aesthetic medicine, an important **spatial characteristic of the light beam is collimation, which is the degree of divergence of the beam's rays**. Clearly, the higher the divergence of the rays, the more difficult it is to collect them in a small spot, which is often necessary for local treatment.

Comparing the area of light spots from a pocket lamp and a laser pointer shows that the laser beam is characterized by a high degree of collimation, manifested by the strict parallelism of its rays. This also allows good optical focusing and, therefore, a large energy density — in other words, a high concentration of energy in a microscopically small volume of matter — as well as the ability to transmit radiation over long distances using light guides.

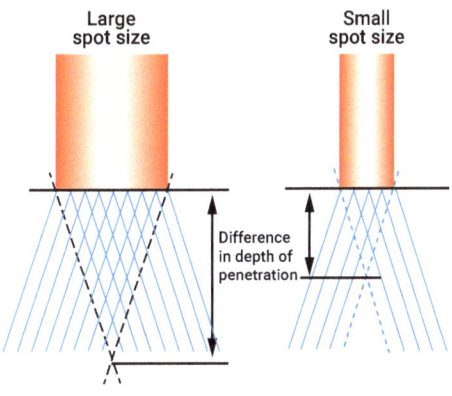

Figure III-1-6. Dependence of the effective penetration depth on the laser spot size

The size of the light spot also determines the effective exposure depth. Since photons are scattered when the laser light interacts with the tissue, this limits the delivery of the energy needed for deep chromophores. If we use a large spot size, we can reduce scattering losses and direct more photons to the target structure, ensuring deeper and more effective delivery of laser energy. However, if a surface effect is required, the spot size should simply be reduced (**Fig. III-1-6**).

Chapter 2
Interaction of laser radiation with the skin

The interaction of the laser beam with the skin follows the laws of physics: laser-emitted light, like all light, can be reflected, scattered, or absorbed, or it can just pass through (**Fig. III-2-1**).

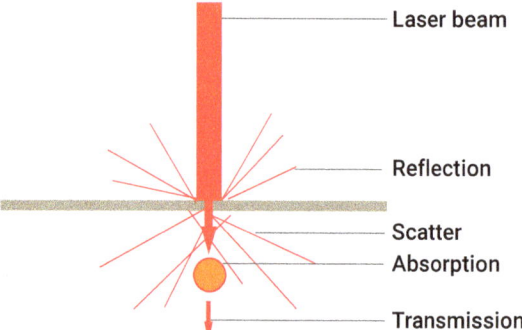

Figure III-2-1. Interaction of laser radiation with the skin

2.1. Laser targets

We can exert a meaningful effect on a substance only if the laser energy is absorbed. Obtaining additional energy by a molecule (transition to an excited state) can serve as a trigger for physicochemical and biological reactions that form the final therapeutic effect. At the same time, each type of electromagnetic field and radiation causes specific photobiological processes, which determine the specificity of their therapeutic effects.

Thus, light-based technologies rely on the specific interaction of electromagnetic radiation of a certain wavelength (photons) with specific substances in the skin capable of absorbing this radiation. These substances, called chromophores, are the main targets of irradiation.

In the case of photodestructive technologies, these chromophores are large structures such as melanin, hemoglobin (oxy- and deoxy-

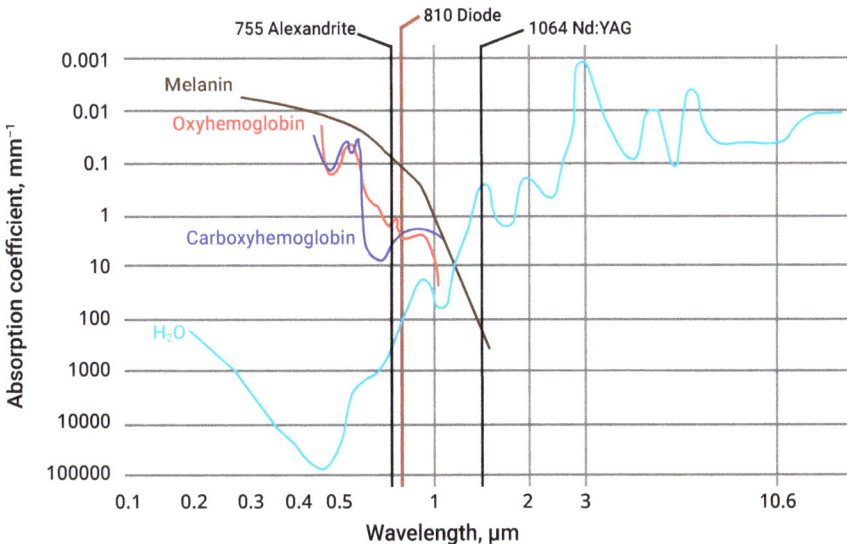

Figure III-2-2. Absorption spectra of laser radiation for different skin chromophores

hemoglobin), water, tattoo pigments, and photosensitizers. Each is characterized by its own absorption spectrum — a curve showing the amount of light absorbed at different wavelengths (**Fig. III-2-2**).

For photobiomodulation, things are much more subtle, but we will talk about that later.

2.2. Laser exposure mechanisms

Further events following the absorption of photons may develop according to different scenarios, but the first stage is always the same: the photons are absorbed by the corresponding chromophores.

In terms of physics, the energy of electromagnetic radiation is converted into other types of energy when interacting with molecules in the body tissues:
- **Chemical energy**, which changes the configuration of electronic bonds in the molecule and its chemical reactivity
- **Thermal energy**, which increases the amplitude of oscillations of the molecule

There are two reasons why the skin heats up when its surface is irradiated:
1. Due to the absorption of light by chromophores (primary)
2. Due to the light scattering in optical inhomogeneities in the epidermis and dermis (secondary)

Even minor heating has serious consequences since tissues can already become damaged at relatively low temperatures — about 42–45 °C (**Table III-2-1**). In some cases, this is exactly what we are trying to achieve: these are classic high-energy laser technologies; in others (low-level laser exposure), we are trying to avoid them.

Table III-2-1. Tissue response to light heating to different temperatures

TEMPERATURE (°C)	BIOLOGICAL EFFECTS
42–45	Structural changes in proteins, breaking of hydrogen bonds, tissue retraction (shrinkage)
45–50	Enzyme inactivation, lipid gelatinization, changes in membrane permeability
50–60	Protein and DNA denaturation, vascular lumen closure
65–80	Denaturation of collagen
100	Water boiling, rupture of vacuoles
100–300	Vaporization (ablation)
200	Denaturation of elastin
100–300	Carbonation (after vaporization)

Depending on the light exposure (energy, pulse duration, and other parameters), the following reactions may occur in the irradiated tissues:
- Photochemical (photobiomodulation)
- Photothermal
- Photoacoustic (photomechanical)

The last two refer to selective and non-selective photodestruction. We discuss photodestruction in the *Lasers in Cosmetic Dermatology & Skincare Practice* book. In this edition, we will consider photobiomodulation.

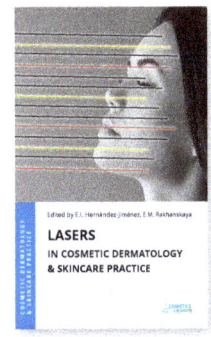

Chapter 3
Photobiomodulation

The term **photobiomodulation** (or **photomodulation**) is used to refer to the technology of skin irradiation with low doses of red and near-IR light (630–950 nm) to modulate (stimulate or inhibit) the functional activity of cells to achieve a positive therapeutic effect.

Why these wavelengths? Light absorption and light scattering in tissues are wavelength-dependent (much higher in the blue region of the spectrum than in the red), and the main tissue chromophores (hemoglobin and melanin) have high absorption bands at wavelengths shorter than 600 nm. Water begins to absorb significantly at wavelengths above 1150 nm. For these reasons, there is a so-called "optical window" covering the red and near-IR bands where the effective light penetration into the tissue is the greatest (see **Fig. III-2-2**). Thus, although blue, green, and yellow light can have a significant effect on cells growing in an optically transparent culture medium, the low-level laser therapy in animals and patients almost exclusively relies on red and near-IR light (630–950 nm) (Hamblin M.R., Demidova T.N., 2006).

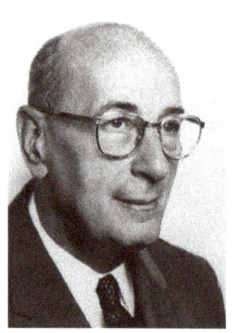

Endre Mester
(1903–1984)

Photobiomodulation was discovered in 1967 through the experiments of the Hungarian scientist Endre Mester (Semmelweis University Budapest, Hungary), who tried to detect the carcinogenic effect of a ruby laser emitting at 694 nm. Mester did not find a carcinogenic effect but did, to his surprise, see a clear increase in hair growth on the shaved areas exposed to radiation.

Further research on the phototherapeutic effect of low-level laser (light*) therapy (LLLT), mainly focused on the wound-healing effect. After the invention of laser diodes, which replaced bulky and expensive lasers, numerous compact devices for photobiomodulation with various types of light pulses emerged. The advantages that these light sources had over lasers — their compactness, their high efficiency that helped minimize heat generation, and the use of a low-voltage power supply — have stimulated the research on photobiomodulation. Now these devices are actively conquering the market of in-home skincare devices.

Currently, LLLT refers to the use of light generated by lasers, or light-emitting diodes with wavelengths of 390–950 nm in continuous or pulsed mode, which have relatively low energy density (0.04–50 J/cm^2) and power (< 100 mW). Wavelengths in the 390–600 nm range are used primarily to correct superficial processes, while longer wavelengths in the 600 to 1000 nm range, which penetrate further, are used to treat more deeply located tissues. It has been noted that wavelengths in the 700 to 750 nm range have limited biochemical activity and are practically unused (Chung H. et al., 2012).

The most frequently used for LLLT are noble gas lasers and semiconductor laser diodes, such as (Hamblin M.R., Demidova T.N., 2006):
- HeNe (632.8 nm)
- Ruby (694 nm)
- Argon (488 and 514 nm)
- Krypton (521, 530, 568, 647 nm)
- Gallium arsenide (GaAs; >760 nm, with a common example of 904 nm) and gallium-aluminum arsenide (GaAlAs; 612–870 nm) semiconductor laser diodes

Another important point that concerns LLLT parameters is biphasic dependence known as the "exposure energy — effect". In contrast to high-energy lasers, for which there will be conditionally linear dependence (that is, the stimulating effect turns into a destructive one depending on the energy), for LLLT, the effect first increases and then

---

* The word "light" reflects the possibility of using not only laser but also light-emitting diodes.

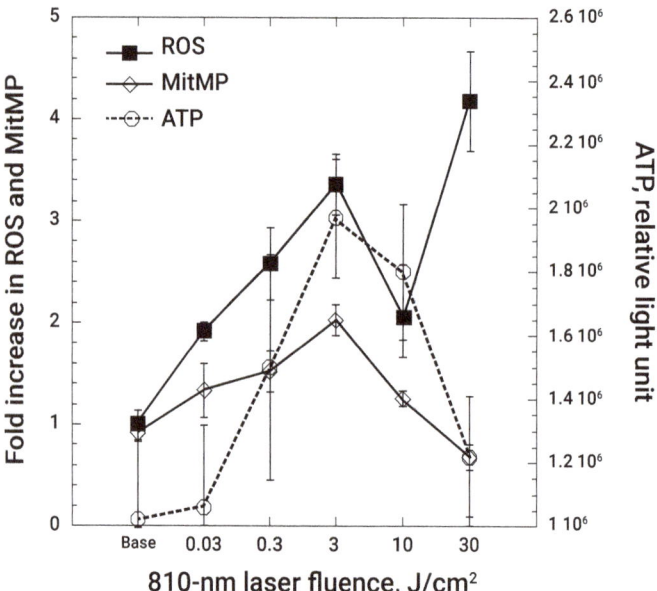

Figure III-3-1. Dependence of LLLT effects — intracellular level of ROS, mitochondrial membrane potential (MitMP), and ATP — on neurons of experimental animals on light energy density (adapted from Huang Y.Y. et al., 2011)

decreases. This is good because it is difficult to provoke irreversible reactions. However, it is also difficult to cause the desired effect, as it is necessary to deliver the exact amount of energy to the chromophore. **Fig. III-3-1** shows the dependence of the LLLT effects — intracellular level of ROS, mitochondrial membrane potential values (an indicator of mitochondrial activity), and ATP — on the neurons of experimental animals on the LLLT energy density (Huang Y.Y. et al., 2011).

3.1. Low laser (light) therapy mechanisms of action

Several hypotheses have been proposed to explain the biophysical and physiological mechanisms underlying the action of LLLT on cells and tissues. Each of these postulates is based on extensive experimental data.

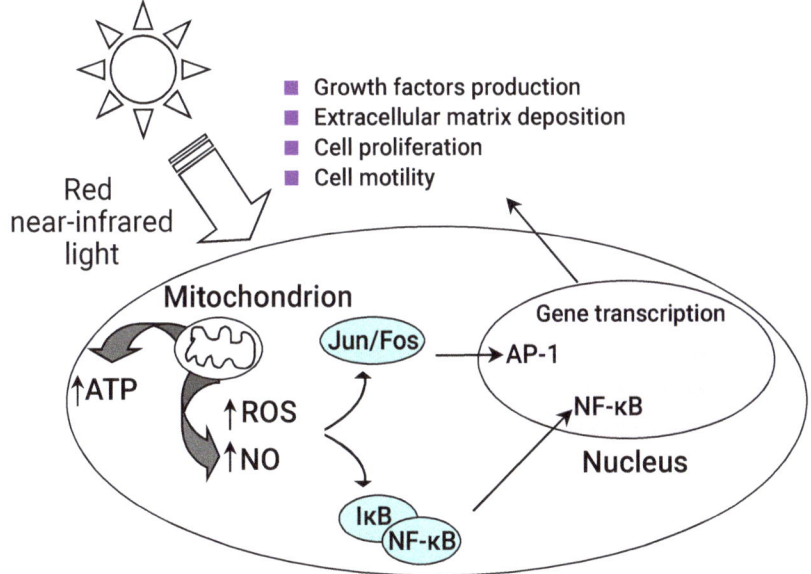

Figure III-3-2. LLLT-induced signaling pathways in the cell (adapted from Photobiological Sciences Online, http://www.photobiology.info)

3.1.1. Mitochondrial hypothesis

In 1988, the photobiologist Tiina Karu proposed the mitochondrial hypothesis, according to which **the mechanism of photomodulation is based on the influence of red and IR light on the mitochondrial respiration, accelerating electron transport along the respiratory chain during oxidative phosphorylation**.

Cytochrome c oxidase, one of the enzymes involved in electron transport, is thought to be the target (**Fig. III-3-2**). The consequences can include:

- Changing the redox state of cytochrome *c* oxidase accelerates the movement of electrons along the respiratory chain and increases ATP production, which enhances metabolic processes in the cell.
- Cytochrome *c* oxidase activity is regulated by humoral factors such as nitric oxide (NO), which inhibits enzymatic activity. Due to the light absorption, NO detaches from the enzyme and thus

increases its activity. In several pathological conditions, NO level can increase, mainly due to macrophage production, which leads to a decrease in ATP production in mitochondria and worsening cell energy supply.
- The assumption that the acceleration of electrons along the respiratory chain can increase the production of superoxide anion, which, in turn, can perform a signaling function in the cell, is being considered.
- There is also the assumption of local heating due to absorbed light and the resulting conformational rearrangements that change the activity of cytochrome *c* oxidase.

The above-described possible processes alter cell activity and trigger secondary reactions associated with the cascades of regulation of the functional state of cells:
- The ATP increase in the cell is a fairly strong regulatory parameter that changes the activity of many enzymes.
- There are transcription factors in the cell that are sensitive to changes in the mitochondrial redox state: nuclear factor kappa B (NF-κB) and activating protein 1 (AP-1). It is the activation of these factors that is associated with the enhancement of protein synthesis in the cell after photostimulation.

Karu's subsequent work showed that the following peak wavelength ranges are most suitable for stimulation of these effects (Karu T.I., Kolyakov S.F., 2005):
- 613.5–623.5 nm
- 667.5–683.7 nm
- 750.7–772.3 nm
- 812.5–846.0 nm

3.1.2. Oxidative stress hypothesis

Besides the action of light on mitochondria, physiological manifestations of irradiation may be related to other processes as well. In 1994, Yuri Vladimirov formulated a hypothesis of three primary mechanisms of LLLT action (with an intensity of no more than 50–100 mW), according to

which laser irradiation can cause three different types of photochemical reactions (each reaction has its own acceptors):
1. Photooxidation of lipids in cell membranes
2. Photoreactivation of the enzyme superoxide dismutase (SOD)
3. Photolysis of nitric oxide (NO) complexes

Due to the increased "release" of ROS, oxidative stress occurs in the cell, forcing it to mobilize its defense and detoxification systems.

3.1.3. Copper hypothesis

We should consider an option of red-light wound healing stimulation by activating the copper-containing tripeptide glycyl-L-histidyl-L-lysine (Cu-GHK). This peptide was discovered by Loren Pickart in 1973. As several investigations on laboratory animals and in *in vitro* studies have shown, the Cu-GHL complex enhances the wound healing process because:
1. It is a powerful anti-inflammatory agent that limits oxidative damage to tissues.
2. It serves as a signaling molecule that promotes tissue repair by activating the removal of damaged proteins and their replacement with normal ones.

As aqueous solutions of copper salts are blue, it is unsurprising that the Cu-GHL intensely absorbs red rays of about 610 nm. Can light enhance the beneficial effects of Cu-GHK on the skin? Huang et al. (2007) tried to answer this question by studying *in vitro* the speed of fibroblast proliferation and collagen production under the combined effect of Cu-GHL and light emitted by red LED (625–635 nm). Cell irradiation (1 J) performed in isolation increased cell viability by 12.5 times. However, combined with Cu-GHK, the secretion of the basic fibroblast growth factor (bFGF) increased by 2.3-fold and the expression of collagen type I matrix RNA increased by 70%.

3.1.4. Thermodynamic hypothesis

According to the generally accepted opinion, each photoinduced process should have its own acceptor (absorber, chromophore) of photons with given energy (in other words, radiation with a certain wavelength). However, an automatic transfer of the "acceptor" model to the therapeutic (biological) action of low-level laser radiation cannot explain some experimental data and clinical observations (Moskvin S.V., 2016). Perhaps this issue should be approached from another angle, considering this radiation as an external factor that triggers physiological reactions.

The first aspect of interest here is that the effect is caused only by the optimal dose of red light. When the dose is decreased or increased in a sufficiently narrow range, the effect decreases or is absent. This is the principal difference between low-intensity red light action and the photobiological phenomena, where the dose dependence has broadly increased. Another surprising fact is the absence of the so-called action spectrum, i.e., specific dependence of the photobiomodulation effect on the light wavelength: the effects occur in the entire spectral range — from 0.337 to 10.6 μm.

These findings allowed Sergei Moskvin to suggest that such effects can be caused by thermodynamic (in fact, thermal) disturbances in intracellular components due to light absorption. Theoretical estimates show that local heating of acceptors by tens of degrees is possible when exposed to laser radiation. Although the process lasts for a very short period (about 10^{-12} s), this is enough for very significant thermodynamic changes, both directly in the target chromophores and in the surrounding regions, leading to pronounced changes in the properties of the molecules and triggering the laser-induced reaction. We should again emphasize that **any intracellular component that actively absorbs a given wavelength can act as an acceptor (chromophore). That is, according to the thermodynamic hypothesis, the initial trigger for the biological action of red light is not the photobiological reaction as such, but the local heating.**

Based on the above arguments, it is evident why the effect is achieved by exposure to **laser** radiation. If the radiation spectrum is comparable to the absorption band of a macromolecule (30 nm or more), such radiation will cause fluctuations in all energy levels, and only weak heating (by fractions of a degree) of the whole molecule will occur. On the contrary, the narrow-spectrum radiation typical for lasers (less than 3 nm) will heat a small area of the macromolecule by dozens of degrees, causing thermodynamic changes sufficient to trigger a further physiological response. Drawing a conditional and obvious analogy, the process can be represented as follows: if a magnifying glass concentrates sunlight at one point, it is possible to set fire to paper, whereas if the entire paper surface is illuminated by scattered light, nothing happens.

This photoinduced change in the "behavior" of macromolecules results in the release of calcium ions from the calcium depot. An increase in the local Ca^{2+} concentration in the cytosol causes numerous calcium-dependent processes inside the cells. Moreover, calcium ions diffuse to neighboring cells and activate them. This spiking mechanism allows the initial local signal to trigger global waves and fluctuations in Ca^{2+} concentrations.

According to the thermodynamic hypothesis, the dose-dependent biphasic effect of laser irradiation is explained by the fact that as the dose increases so does the local temperature, which causes the release of Ca^{2+}. As soon as the amount of Ca^{2+} in the cytosol begins to exceed a certain critical level, mechanisms of pumping Ca^{2+} into calcium depots are activated and the effect disappears.

Primary photobiological reactions cause a wide variety of biochemical and physiological responses, which are a complex of secondary adaptation and compensatory reactions aimed at the recovery of the organism:
- Activation of cell metabolism and increase of cells' functional activity
- Stimulation of reparative processes
- Anti-inflammatory effect
- Activation of skin blood circulation and increase in blood supply to tissues
- Analgesic effect
- Immunostimulating effect
- Reflexogenic effect on the functional activity of various organs and systems

The proposed scheme of development of biological effects from laser exposure according to the thermodynamic hypothesis is shown in **Fig. III-3-3**.

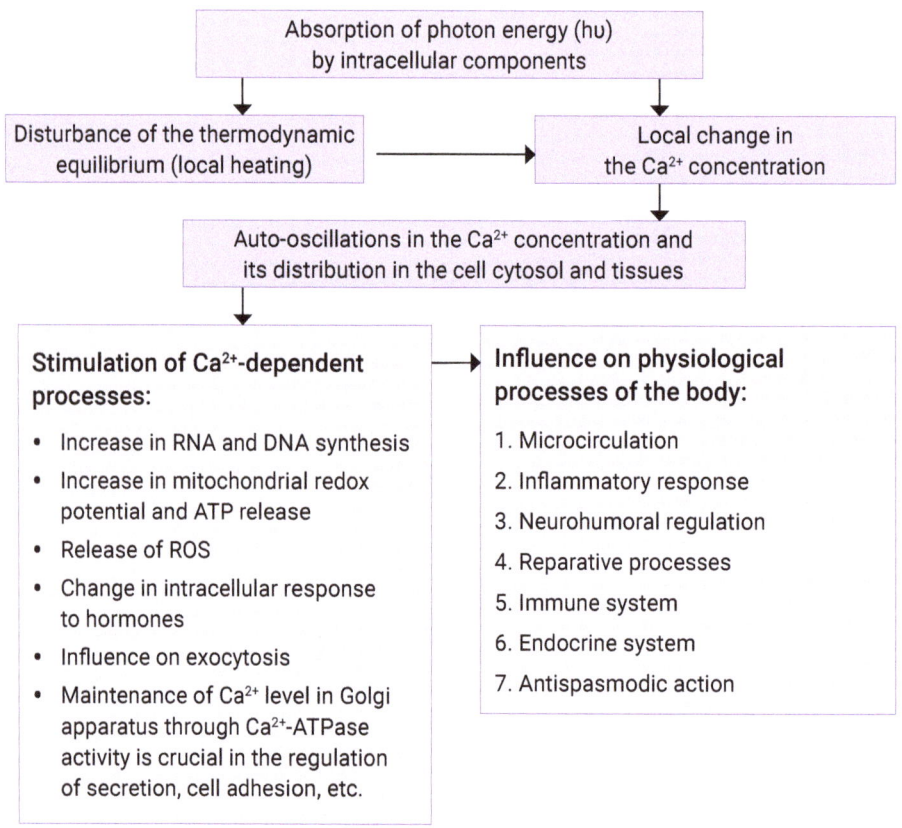

Figure III-3-3. Sequence of development of laser exposure-induced biological effects (according to Moskvin's thermodynamic hypothesis)

3.2. Clinical effects and therapeutic applications

Before we move on to the possibilities of photobiomodulation in medicine and skincare, we would like to dwell on the following issue.

The fact is that, despite the inspiring laboratory studies of LLLT and its fairly wide use in both professional and home-based procedures, in practice, not everything is as smooth as it could be. There are several reasons for this variability, according to Avci P. et al. (2013).

First, despite decades of study and application of LLLT, the mechanisms of its action are still not completely understood. Consequently, it is impossible to choose optimal parameters of exposure and to predict the effects of therapy. As noted above, in the case of LLLT, fine-tuning is very important; even a small deviation of parameters can lead to the suppression rather than stimulation of some processes.

Second, there are significant differences in the parameters used by different scientists and practitioners — wavelength, energy density or power, exposure mode, coherence, contact or non-contact application, exposure time and pattern, number of treatments, etc. — which create difficulties in comparing and predicting results. Many of the data are obtained under "ideal" conditions, and in practice, to achieve them, strict requirements need to be followed, such as the distance from the light source to the skin. Even a minimal offset from the manufacturer's intended distance will have a significant effect on the results.

It is perhaps because of these ambiguities that many of the published studies on LLLT have yielded negative outcomes. In practice, specialists and patients are not always satisfied with the treatment results. This may also be due to improper preparation of the patient's skin prior to LLLT application, such as insufficient removal of makeup and oily residues that may interfere with light penetration and failure to consider the effects of skin pigmentation.

This is why one of the most important prerequisites for obtaining the desired effects is using certified devices and working with them exactly according to the manual. This applies to professional devices and widespread LED masks, the efficiency of which is already somewhat lower than that of laser diode devices.

We will not go into the specifics of their use within this book, because they will vary greatly from manufacturer to manufacturer, although we wish to note again that following the recommendations in the manual is the key to obtaining results from a particular device. In addition, in all cases, a series of treatments is mandatory to get the intended effect.

In clinical practice, red and near-IR light is most often used for the treatment of subacute and chronic inflammatory lesions and subcutaneous tissue disorders (atopic dermatitis, acne, rosacea, psoriasis, etc.), chronic wounds and trophic ulcers, burns and frostbite, itching dermatosis, furunculosis, and thymus-dependent immunodeficiency conditions.

The anti-inflammatory effect, the acceleration of damaged tissue regeneration, and improvement of their blood supply under laser red light observed in clinical practice can be associated with the following impacts (Machneva T.V. et al., 2012; Hartmann D.D. et al., 2021):

1. Increased phagocyte activity
2. Increased cell proliferation
3. Improvement of blood circulation through the vascular bed due to vasodilation

Immune disorders are observed in many skin diseases. Radiation-induced phagocyte activation is manifested by a two- or three-fold increase in the release of ROS (superoxide, hydrogen peroxide, hypochlorite) and nitric oxide (NO): phagocytes turn into a kind of "bombers", throwing shells at enemy objects. Foreign cells (bacteria, fungi, body's own "sick" cells) are broken into pieces and are absorbed by immunocytes through phagocytosis. NO-triggered vasodilation and blood flow to the site of "battle" take place. The essence of phagocyte activation is as follows. Under laser light, in the presence of photosensitizers (hematoporphyrin or phthalocyanine), free radical oxidation of lipids can be initiated in cell membranes, which leads to the entry of Ca^{2+} into the cell. An increase in the intracellular Ca^{2+} level serves as a signal to trigger many processes, particularly an increase in the number of cell receptors. The effect of cell pre-stimulation is mainly determined by the concentration of photosensitizers in the cell membranes, which, in turn, depends on the patient's condition. Healthy people may have no photosensitizers in the cell membranes, and there is no effect of phagocyte pre-stimulation. For unhealthy people, there could be a photosensitizer in the cell membranes, and the pre-stimulation is well pronounced. **Pre-stimulation of phagocytes is mainly observed due to blood irradiation.**

When treating certain skin diseases, in addition to local laser therapy, **blood irradiation** is performed **in an invasive or non-invasive manner**. The invasive method consists of the venipuncture (venesection) in the radial vein, blood intake of 500–750 ml, and laser irradiation, followed by reinfusion of irradiated blood. The procedure is performed every six months with 30-minute exposure. In the non-invasive method, the laser beam is brought to the projection of the radial vein. The patient clenches and unclenches the fist. As a result, 70% of the blood is irradiated within 30 minutes. The method is painless, does not require special conditions, and involves continuous and pulsed laser irradiation. Blood irradiation is performed for allergic dermatoses (atopic dermatitis, chronic eczema, recurrent urticaria), psoriasis, pyoderma, and vasculitis.

In both local skin irradiation and intravenous blood irradiation, LLLT has an immunomodulatory effect: dysglobulinemia is eliminated, phagocytosis activity increases, apoptosis is normalized, and the neuroendocrine system is activated.

The effect of LLLT on fibroblasts has also been studied, which is important for both skin rejuvenation and scar repair processes. The first studies on animals in this field were conducted as early as 1987, showing an increase in the production of procollagen, collagen, fibroblast basic growth factor (bFGF), as well as fibroblast proliferation in response to 633-nm radiation exposure, in both *in vitro* and *in vivo* conditions (Abergel R.P. et al., 1987). In later experiments on humans, the effect on matrix metalloproteinases (MMPs) and their tissue inhibitors (TIMPs; enzymes responsible for the destruction of the dermal matrix), as well as other agents that characterize the immune status and structural integrity of the skin (Lee S.Y. et al., 2007a), was shown. As a part of this study, Lee S.Y. et al. (2007a) analyzed data on 76 volunteers (predominantly women aged 35–55 with skin phototypes III and IV) with facial wrinkles. The participants were randomly divided into four groups. Depending on the group, one side of the person's face was irradiated with an LED source: either 830 nm only, 633 nm only, or a combination of 830 and 633 nm, or a "placebo" lamp two times a week for four weeks. Objective skin analysis showed a significant reduction in wrinkle expression (up to 36%) and an increase in skin elasticity (up to 19%) compared to the baseline on the treated side of the face in all three experimental groups.

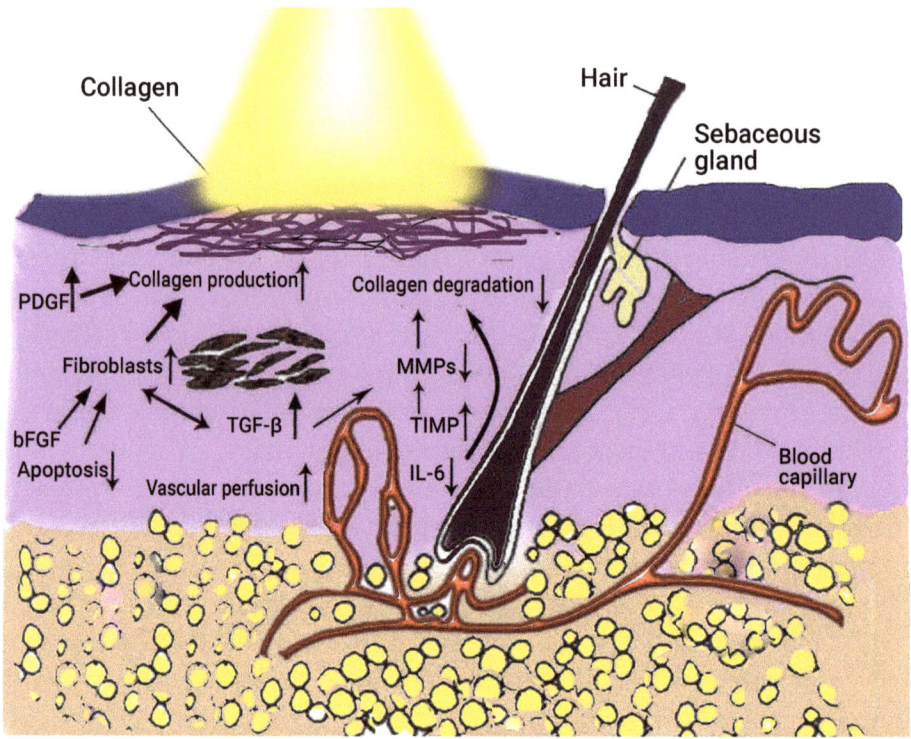

Figure III-3-4. Effects of LLLT that may be responsible for its rejuvenating and regenerative properties (adapted from Avci P. et al., 2013)

Biopsies taken from the treated areas showed a marked increase in collagen and elastin fibers, fibroblast activity, TIMP-1 and TIMP-2 levels, IL-1β and TNF-α mRNA early expression, ICAM-1 and connexin 43 (Cx43) (responsible for intercellular contacts), along with a decrease in proinflammatory IL-6 (**Fig. III-3-4**) (Avci P. et al., 2013). The pro-inflammatory cytokines IL-1β and TNF-α are thought to be involved in wound healing and promote collagen synthesis. They also activate MMP, so an increase in their levels in the early period may indicate MMP activation to break down photodamaged collagen. After the necessary work is done, however, they are inhibited by TIMP so that fibroblasts can quietly produce new collagen and elastin (Lee S.Y. et al., 2007a).

Interesting results were obtained in a study of the responses of human dermal fibroblast subpopulations to LLLT of different wavelengths

(450, 490, 530, 590, 650, and 850 nm) (Mignon C. et al., 2018). The work was performed to determine the radiation parameters that would have a high therapeutic potential for slowing down skin aging and treating chronic wounds. It was established that LLLT at 450, 490, and 530 nm inhibited fibroblast activity, 590-nm treatment had no significant effect, and 850-nm one demonstrated a significant stimulating effect on fibroblasts. This knowledge can be used both to stimulate collagen formation and to inhibit it, for example, in preventing hypertrophic scars (although there remains the question of penetration of shorter-wavelength radiation into the deeper layers of the skin).

Low-level laser radiation also has **an analgesic effect due to decreased sensitivity of the skin receptors, increased pain threshold, and stimulation of opioid receptors**. At the same time, there is a mild sedative effect. The combination of sedative and analgesic effects is especially important when the disease is accompanied by itching (allergic dermatosis, pruritic dermatosis, lichen planus).

3.3. Indications and applications in skincare

3.3.1. Age-related skin changes

The rejuvenating effect of photobiomodulation is due to the action of red and IR light, namely stimulating the proliferation of keratinocytes and fibroblasts, increasing their activity, and with it strengthening the extracellular matrix, anti-inflammatory effect (inflammaging — aging due to inflammation — one of the main factors accelerating the appearance of signs of aging skin) and improving microcirculation.

Weiss R.A. et al. (2005a) studied the effect of 590-nm LLLT for treating age-related changes. The study involved 90 people with signs of mild to moderate facial photoaging. All participants received eight LLLT sessions for four weeks with different pulse sequences and energy density of 0.1 J/cm. The outcome was highly favorable: more than 90% of patients had improved skin condition in at least one parameter of the Fitzpatrick photoaging scale, and 65% of patients demonstrated an overall improvement in facial texture, reduction in fine lines, background erythema, and pigmentation. Results peaked 4–6 months after completing the eight treatments (Weiss R.A. et al., 2005a). However, it should be noted that, given the neutral effect of 590-nm LLLT on fibroblasts (although it is incorrect to compare *in vivo* and *in vitro* studies due to the very different energy of light exposure that cells in culture and living tissue receive), the effect may be related not only to the effect on fibroblasts, but also to the anti-inflammatory effect of this spectrum of radiation (Lan C.C. et al., 2015; Mignon C. et al., 2018).

Rejuvenating effects of LLLT were also shown in a split-face study conducted by Barolet D. et al. (2009) as a part of which one half of the face was treated, the other was not (660-nm LLLT with 12 treatments for one month, energy density of 4 J/cm^2, energy flux density of 50 mW/cm^2). Histological control confirmed a 35% increase in procollagen-1 and an 18% decrease in MMPs.

3.3.2. Skin recovery

The LLLT-assisted rejuvenating effect is based on stimulating the proliferation and activity of keratinocytes and fibroblasts, anti-inflammatory action, and improvement of microcirculation. The analgesic effect of LLLT will also contribute here.

All these effects might be useful in treating damaged skin. The study conducted by Weiss R.A. et al. (2005b) with 600 patients showed that LLLT (590 nm, 0.1 J/cm^2) accelerated the recovery and erythema reduction after high-energy physical treatments (IPL, PDL- and potassium-titanyl-phosphate (KTP) lasers, ablative lasers, and RF). The erythema reduction can be attributed to the anti-inflammatory effects of LLLT.

3.3.3. Acne

A combination of red and blue light is recommended for treating acne-prone skin (Sadick N.S., 2008). The red light of 630-nm wavelength causes an anti-inflammatory effect and inhibits sebum production. The blue light gives the expected antiseptic effect. In addition, *C. acnes* synthesize porphyrins that, when absorbed by blue light (407–420 nm), are excited, followed by the release of ROS, which leads to irreversible membrane damage and death of the bacterial cell. Unfortunately, blue light cannot penetrate the skin deeply enough to kill all the bacteria settled in the sebaceous glands. Nevertheless, blue light (415 nm) has been shown to suppress sebocyte proliferation (Jung Y.R. et al., 2015).

In addition, LLLT in the IR range (820 nm) also provides an anti-inflammatory effect, penetrating as deeply as possible, modulating cytokine release from macrophages, regulating keratinocyte proliferation, eliminating hyperkeratosis, and improving blood flow (Li W.H. et al., 2018). Therefore, the best effects of LLLT are seen in inflammatory rather than comedonal acne.

In many cases, LLLT is not used as the main treatment, but as an adjunctive treatment in addition to standard therapy. However, as a monomethod, it helps to maintain remission.

3.3.4. Pigmentation disorders: vitiligo and pigment lesions

In 1982, a positive effect of LLLT on catecholamine synthesis in scleroderma and vitiligo was shown. In the study with 18 vitiligo patients, after 6–8 months of treatment with low-energy HeNe laser (633 nm, 25 mW/cm^2) there was a noticeable repigmentation in 64% of participants, while the remaining 34% had some follicular repigmentation (Mandel A.S., Dunaeva L.P., 1982; Mandel A.S. et al., 1997). Since then, LLLT has been widely used as an alternative treatment for vitiligo patients, although it does not result in complete recovery (Avci P. et al., 2013). This effect is associated with a direct activating effect on melanocytes and their adhesion to the matrix and neuro-regenerative action (for segmental vitiligo), as well as increased blood circulation and reduced inflammation.

The depigmenting LLLT effect was found unexpectedly in a study concerning acne treatment with blue and red light (Lee S.Y. et al., 2007b). A combination of blue (415 ± 5 nm, energy flux density of 40 mW/cm^2, energy density of 48 J/cm^2) and red (633 ± 6 nm, 80 mW/cm^2, 96 J/cm^2) light resulted in an overall reduction in melanin levels which was attributed to red light. However, there has been little further research on this matter. One could speculate that since different parameters are used to treat vitiligo and acne, the different effects of red light on the same tissue could be due to the biphasic LLLT action. Again, this brings us back to the ambiguity of therapy effects due to using different exposure parameters. It is important to follow the manufacturer's recommendations, but in any case, we should be prepared for surprises.

3.3.5. Atopic dermatitis and psoriasis

We will not elaborate on these diseases, as they are primarily dermatological issues (for details, see the *Dry Skin, Atopic Dermatitis and Psoriasis in Cosmetic Dermatology & Skincare Practice* book). But let us say that LLLT is actively used as an adjunctive therapy for treating these diseases. Improvement is achieved through the immunomodulatory, anti-inflammatory, sedative, and analgesic effects (Kemény L. et al., 2019).

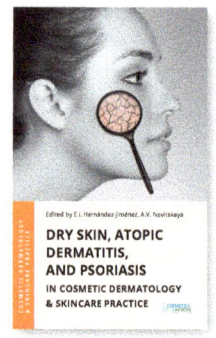

3.3.6. Alopecia

The possibility of stimulating hair growth using laser radiation initiated the development of photobiomodulation. Recall that, back in 1967, Endre Mester, who tried to detect the carcinogenic effect of a Ruby laser emitting red light of 694 nm, instead found a clear increase in hair growth on shaved areas exposed to radiation. The same effect has been noted by many specialists practicing laser and IPL epilation: if the supplied energy is insufficient, instead of epilation, we observe paradoxical hypertrichosis. The incidence of this effect, according to various data sources, ranges from 0.6% to 10%. It is assumed that heat insufficient for the thermolysis of hair follicles may cause the proliferation and differentiation of follicular stem cells by increasing the levels of heat shock proteins such as HSP27. This protein plays a role in regulating cell growth and differentiation (hair follicles and vessels), leading to, among other effects, the degeneration of downy hair into terminal ones. Among other observed impacts, an increase in the anagen phase, reentry into anagen from telogen, and prevention of premature catagen development are noted (Avci P. et al., 2014).

Special devices in the form of helmets and laser combs have been developed to irradiate the scalp. LLLT in the 630–660-nm spectral range is mainly used to enhance hair growth in different types of alopecia (androgenetic, telogenic, etc.). The effects are seen after a long course of treatment. The U.S. Food and Drug Administration approved using low-intensity laser treatment with a laser comb for treating androgenetic alopecia in men and women (in 2007 and 2011, respectively).

3.3.7. Local fat deposits

In 2002, the effect of low-intensity laser red light (635 nm) on abdominal fat was studied in humans (Neira R. et al., 2002). The nuclear magnetic resonance (NMR) spectroscopy showed that, after laser irradiation, there was a blurring of contours of adipose tissue and changes in fibrous bands were observed. Scanning and transmission electron microscopy demonstrated the destruction of adipocyte membranes as laser exposure duration increased. The authors further noted that after 4-min light exposure 80% of the fat was released into the intercellular space, and after 6-min exposure, no fat remained in the cells (**Fig. III-3-5**). Electron microscopy revealed the appearance of temporary pores in cells induced by laser irradiation, through which fat was released from the cells. This work opened the prospect of using red light to influence abdominal fat (so-called cold laser lipolysis).

Subsequent studies demonstrated a fairly rapid return of adipocytes to their previous shape (while maintaining the previous lifestyle), because, unlike high-energy lipodestruction treatment, LLLT does not destroy adipocytes — neither apoptosis nor necrosis is achieved. The most pronounced effect of the cold lipo laser is

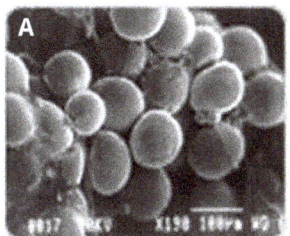 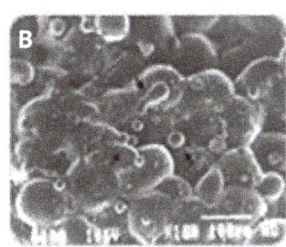 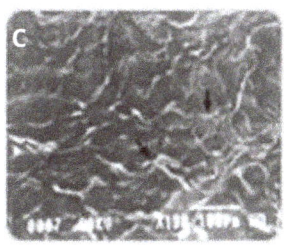

Figure III-3-5. Destruction of adipocytes under low-intensity laser red light: A — before irradiation; B — after 4-min irradiation; C — after 6-min irradiation (adapted from Neira R. et al., 2002)

observed in the weeks following the procedure; however, in three months, there is a recovery of half of the lost volume. Conversely, after cryolipolysis, this is the time when the first effects emerge, but persist for a long time (Kennedy J. et al., 2015).

Thus, LLLT can be used to shape the body, but it is necessary to adequately assess its capabilities. Nonetheless, according to the results of surveys and patients' self-assessments, they are quite satisfied with the results of cold laser lipolysis, as well as the comfort and painlessness of the treatment (Kennedy J. et al., 2015).

In some cases, there can be opposite effects. For example, in the study condcuted by Jankowski M. et al. (2017), a paradoxical increase in the thickness of the fat occurred in eight out of 17 patients after six LLLT procedures (650 nm, surface flux density of 9.14 mW/cm^2, energy density per session of 7.5 J/cm^2). Although the authors did not guarantee that all participants followed the same lifestyle and exercise regime, they did warn about the risk of such an effect.

3.4. Contraindications

The following contraindications are defined for photobiomodulation (Navratil L., Kymplova J., 2002):
- Neoplasms
- Histologically detected malignant carcinomain in anamnesis
- Hyperthermia
- In hyperthyroidism — irradiation of the neck area
- Photopathology (porphyria, taking photosensitizers)
- Active tuberculosis
- Epilepsy
- Exposure to the abdomen during pregnancy
- Hypertension of stages II–III
- Blood diseases

Afterword

In this book, we have compiled scientifically validated information on the principles and therapeutic possibilities of low-energy microcurrent, ultrasound and LED therapy. As we can see, despite the differences in physical nature and engineering, the clinical results of these procedures are in many ways similar — they help to "rejuvenate, restore, revitalize" the skin. To get predictable results, you need to know how they work. Our book will help you better understand these methods, and with this new knowledge you will be able to implement and optimize their use in your practice.

References

Abergel R.P., Lyons R.F., Castel J.C. et al. Biostimulation of wound healing by lasers: experimental approaches in animal models and in fibroblast cultures. J Dermatol Surg Oncol 1987; 13(2): 127–133.

Abramson H.A., Gorin M.H. Skin reactions, IX: the electrophoretic demonstration of the patent pores of the living human skin; its relation to the charge of the skin. Phys Chem 1940; 44: 1094–1102.

Arjunan K.P., Clyne A.M. a nitric oxide producing pin-to-hole spark discharge plasma enhances endothelial cell proliferation and migration. Plasma Med 2011a; 1(3–4): 279–293.

Arjunan K.P., Clyne A.M. Hydroxyl radical and hydrogen peroxide are primarily responsible for dielectric barrier discharge plasma-induced angiogenesis. Plasma Process Polym 2011b; 8: 1154–1164.

Avci P., Gupta A., Sadasivam M. et al. Low-level laser (light) therapy (LLLT) in skin: stimulating, healing, restoring. Semin Cutan Med Surg 2013; 32(1): 41–52.

Avci P., Gupta G.K., Clark J. et al. Low-level laser (light) therapy (LLLT) for treatment of hair loss. Lasers Surg Med 2014; 46(2): 144–151.

Bakhovets N.V. Hardware Cosmetology. Microcurrent Therapy. SPb.: Ayuna, 2019a.

Bakhovets N.V. Hardware Cosmetology. Ultrasonic Therapy. SPb: Ayuna, 2019b.

Barolet D., Roberge C.J., Auger F.A. et al. Regulation of skin collagen metabolism *in vitro* using a pulsed 660 nm LED light source: clinical correlation with a single-blinded study. J Invest Dermatol 2009; 129(12): 2751–2759.

Cheng N., Van Hoof H., Bockx E. et al. The effects of electric currents on ATP generation, protein synthesis, and membrane transport of rat skin. Clin Orthop Relat Res 1982; (171): 264–272.

Choi J.H., Lee H.W., Lee J.K. et al. Low-temperature atmospheric plasma increases the expression of anti-aging genes of skin cells without causing cellular damages. Arch Dermatol Res 2013; 305(2): 133–140.

Choi J.H., Song Y.S., Song K. et al. Skin renewal activity of non-thermal plasma through the activation of β-catenin in keratinocytes. Sci Rep 2017; 7(1): 6146.

Chung H., Dai T., Sharma S.K. et al. The nuts and bolts of low-level laser (light) therapy. Ann Biomed Eng 2012; 40(2): 516–533.

Daftardar S., Neupane R., Boddu Sai H.S. et al. Advances in ultrasound-mediated transdermal drug delivery. Curr Pharm Des. 2019; 25(4): 413–423.

Da Silva C.M., de Mello Pinto M.V., Barbosa L.G. et al. Effect of ultrasound and hyaluronidase on gynoid lipodystrophy type II — an ultrasonography study. J Cosmet Laser Ther 2013; 15(4): 231–236.

Foster K.W., Moy R.L., Fincher E.F. Advances in plasma skin regeneration. J Cosmet Dermatol 2008; 7(3): 169–179.

Graves D.B. Mechanisms of Plasma Medicine: Coupling Plasma Physics, Biochemistry and Biology. IEEE Trans Radiat Plasma Med Sci 2017; 1(4): 281–292.

Gulyaev A.A. The use of ultrasound in the practice of a specialist in body contouring. Apparatus Cosmetology and Physical Therapy 2016; 1–2: 182–185.

Hamblin M.R., Demidova T.N. Mechanisms of low level light therapy. SPIE BiOS 2006; 6140: 614001.

Hartmann D.D., Martins R.P., Silva T.C.D. et al. Oxidative stress is involved in LLLT mechanism of action on skin healing in rats. Braz J Med Biol Res 2021; 54(6): e10293.

Huang P.J., Huang Y.C., Su M.F. et al. In vitro observations on the influence of copper peptide aids for the LED photoirradiation of fibroblast collagen synthesis. Photomed Laser Surg. 2007; 25(3): 183–190.

Huang Y.Y., Sharma S.K., Carroll J., Hamblin M.R. Biphasic dose response in low level light therapy — an update. Dose Response 2011; 9(4): 602–618.

Isbary G., Heinlin J., Shimizu T. et al. Successful and safe use of 2 min cold atmospheric argon plasma in chronic wounds: results of a randomized controlled trial. Br J Dermatol 2012; 167(2): 404–410.

Jankowski M., Gawrych M., Adamska U. et al. Low-level laser therapy (LLLT) does not reduce subcutaneous adipose tissue by local adipocyte injury but rather by modulation of systemic lipid metabolism. Lasers Med Sci 2017; 32(2): 475–479.

Jung Y.R., Kim S.J., Sohn K.C. et al. Regulation of lipid production by light-emitting diodes in human sebocytes. Arch Dermatol Res 2015; 307(3): 265–273.

Karu T.I., Kolyakov S.F. Exact action spectra for cellular responses relevant to phototherapy. Photomed Laser Surg 2005; 23(4): 355–361.

Kemény L., Varga E., Novak Z. Advances in phototherapy for psoriasis and atopic dermatitis. Expert Rev Clin Immunol 2019; 15(11): 1205–1214.

Kennedy J., Verne S., Griffith R. et al. Non-invasive subcutaneous fat reduction: a review. J Eur Acad Dermatol Venereol 2015; 29(9): 1679–1688.

Kong M.G., Kroesen G., Morfill G. et al. Plasma medicine: an introductory review. New J Phys 2009; 11(115012): 1–35.

Kos S., Blagus T., Cemazar M. et al. Safety aspects of atmospheric pressure helium plasma jet operation on skin: In vivo study on mouse skin. PLoS One 2017; 12(4): e0174966.

Lan C.C., Ho P.Y., Wu C.S. et al. LED 590 nm photomodulation reduces UVA-induced metalloproteinase-1 expression via upregulation of antioxidant enzyme catalase. J Dermatol Sci 2015; 78(2): 125–132.

Lee O.J., Ju H.W., Khang G. et al. An experimental burn wound-healing study of non-thermal atmospheric pressure microplasma jet arrays. J Tissue Eng Regen Med 2016; 10(4): 348–357.

Lee S.Y., Park K.H., Choi J.W. et al. a prospective, randomized, placebo-controlled, double-blinded, and split-face clinical study on LED phototherapy for skin rejuvenation: clinical, profilometric, histologic, ultrastructural, and biochemical evaluations and comparison of three different treatment settings. J Photochem Photobiol B 2007a; 88(1): 51–67.

Lee S.Y., You C.E., Park M.Y. Blue and red light combination LED phototherapy for acne vulgaris in patients with skin phototype IV. Lasers Surg Med 2007b; 39(2): 180–188.

Levin M., Pezzulo G., Finkelstein J.M. Endogenous bioelectric signaling networks: exploiting voltage gradients for control of growth and form. Annu Rev Biomed Eng 2017; 19: 353–387.

Li W.H., Fassih A., Binner C. et al. Low-level red LED light inhibits hyperkeratinization and inflammation induced by unsaturated fatty acid in an in vitro model mimicking acne. Lasers Surg Med 2018; 50(2): 158–165.

Machneva T.V., Kosmacheva N.V., Vladimirov Y.A., Osipov A.N. The effect of low power laser radiation of blue, green, and red ranges on free radical processes in blood of rats with experimental endotoxic shock. Biomed Khim 2013; 59(4): 237–246.

Maeshige N., Terashi H., Aoyama M. et al. Effect of ultrasound irradiation on α-SMA and TGF-β1 expression in human fibroblasts. Kobe J Med Sci 2011; 56(6): E242–E252.

Mandel A.S., Dunaeva L.P. Effect of laser therapy on blood levels of serotonin and dopamine scleroderma patients. Vestn Dermatol Venerol 1982; 8: 13–17.

Mandel A.S., Haberman H.F., Pawlowski D., Goldstein E. Non PUVA nonsurgical therapies for vitiligo. Clin Dermatol 1997; 15(6): 907–919.

McMakin C., Gregory W., Phillips T. Cytokine changes with microcurrent treatment of fibromyalgia associated with cervical spine trauma. J Bodyw Mov Ther 2005; 9(3): 169–176.

Mignon C., Uzunbajakava N.E., Castellano-Pellicena I. et al. Differential response of human dermal fibroblast subpopulations to visible and near-infrared light: potential of photobiomodulation for addressing cutaneous conditions. Lasers Surg Med 2018; 50(8): 859–882.

Moskvin S.V. Fundamentals of laser therapy. Triad Pub, 2016.

Navratil L., Kymplova J. Contraindications in noninvasive laser therapy: truth and fiction. J Clin Laser Med Surg 2002; 20(6): 341–343.

Neira R., Arroyave J., Ramirez H. et al. Fat liquefaction: effect of low-level laser energy on adipose tissue. Plast Reconstr Surg 2002; 110(3): 912–922; discussion 923–925.

Polat B.E., Hart D., Langer R., Blankschtein D. Ultrasound-mediated transdermal drug delivery: mechanisms, scope, and emerging trends. J Control Release. 2011; 152(3): 330–348.

Rich K.T., Hoerig C.L., Rao M.B., Mast T.D. Relations between acoustic cavitation and skin resistance during intermediate- and high-frequency sonophoresis. J Control Release 2014; 194: 266–277.

Sadick N.S. Handheld LED array device in the treatment of acne vulgaris. J Drugs Dermatol 2008; 7(4): 347–350.

Samuels J., Weingarten M., Margolis D. et al. Low-frequency (<100 kHz), low-intensity (<100 mW/cm^2) ultrasound to treat venous ulcers: a human study and in vitro experiments. J Acoust Soc Am 2013; 134(2): 1541–1547.

Sheptiy O.V., Generalova T.V. Plasma technology in cosmetology and dermatology: new opportunities and prospects for use. Cosmetics and Medicine 2018; 1: 47–55.

Shimizu K., Hayashida K., Blajan M. Novel method to improve transdermal drug delivery by atmospheric microplasma irradiation. Biointerphases 2015; 10(2): 029517.

Tawfik M.A., Tadros M.I., Mohamed M.I., Nageeb El-Helaly S. Low-frequency versus high-frequency ultrasound-mediated transdermal delivery of agomelatine-loaded invasomes: development, optimization and in-vivo pharmacokinetic sssessment. Int J Nanomed 2020;15: 8893-8910.

Tiede R., Hirschberg J., Daeschlei G. et al. Plasma applications: a dermatological view. Contrib Plasma Phys 2014; 54(2): 118–130.

Weiss R.A., McDaniel D.H., Geronemus R.G., Weiss M.A. Clinical trial of a novel nonthermal LED array for reversal of photoaging: clinical, histologic, and surface profilometric results. Lasers Surg Med 2005a; 36(2): 85–91

Weiss R.A., McDaniel D.H., Geronemus R.G. et al. Clinical experience with light-emitting diode (LED) photomodulation. Dermatol Surg 2005b; 31(9 Pt 2): 1199–1205.

www.ingramcontent.com/pod-product-compliance
Lightning Source LLC
LaVergne TN
LVHW050310040526
837301LV00003B/33